Psychology Revivals

Nervous Breakdown

Originally published in 1934, excerpts from the original preface read: "A Nervous breakdown is a terrifying experience. When it occurs, the patient, his family, and often his friends are panic-stricken. No one knows just what to do with the patient, and the patient is incapable of helping himself. ... What should be done? If you think you have a nervous breakdown, it is your first duty to consult a competent and reputable physician, preferably your family doctor, and get a thorough and complete physical examination. If you cannot find any evidence of physical or organic disease, ask your doctor to recommend a reputable psychiatrist or medical psychologist. ...This is a compact manual of help and self-help." Today this book can be read and enjoyed in its historical context.

Nervous Breakdown

Its cause and cure

W.B. Wolfe

Routledge
Taylor & Francis Group
LONDON AND NEW YORK

First published in 1934
by Routledge & Kegan Paul Ltd

This edition first published in 2015 by Routledge
4 Park Square, Milton Park, Abingdon, Oxon OX14 4RN
605 Third Avenue, New York, NY 10017

Routledge is an imprint of the Taylor & Francis Group, an informa business

Publisher's Note

The publisher has gone to great lengths to ensure the quality of this reprint but points out that some imperfections in the original copies may be apparent.

Disclaimer

The publisher has made every effort to trace copyright holders and welcomes correspondence from those they have been unable to contact.

ISBN: 978-1-138-93071-1 (hbk)
ISBN: 978-1-315-68026-2 (ebk)

NERVOUS BREAKDOWN

Its Cause and Cure

BY

W. B. WOLFE, M.D.

LONDON

ROUTLEDGE & KEGAN PAUL LTD

BROADWAY HOUSE: 68-74 CARTER LANE, E.C.4

First published in England 1934
Second impression 1936
Third impression 1949

PRINTED IN GREAT BRITAIN BY
LUND HUMPHRIES
LONDON · BRADFORD

TO

MEN AND WOMEN
IN PERPLEXITY

CONTENTS

justments of university life. Challenged by the threat of being "sent down" from his university, he attempts suicide as a means of evading an intolerable admission of failure; is rescued, but suffers a nervous breakdown.—Social Breakdown: *The case of Ruth G., a young American woman, the victim not only of her mother's social aspirations, but also of a childhood of parental coddling and pampering. She found marriage to a Harvard professor an intolerable betrayal of her romantic ideals. This is the story of a self-appointed princess who eventually finds happiness in hard work.*

CHAPTER FOUR

Sexual Breakdowns—Sexual Ignorance: *The case of Luella D. is the story of a young woman whose nervous breakdown was the immediate result of abject ignorance of sexual hygiene. Marriage was the critical situation, the ignorance of her husband a contributing factor. Enlightenment of both partners effects the cure.*—About Masturbation: *The case of Warren O. illustrates a common type of nervous breakdown associated with worry and remorse over the practice of masturbation. Here the breakdown was a defensive measure designed to forestall a critical test of virility.* —Masculine Protest: *The case of Gladys T., an American woman, is characteristic of many women. She based her sense of "face" on her "sex appeal"—and lost. She had to save her "face" by being ill until she discovered latent personality assets during her psychological re-education.*—Romantic Breakdown: *The case of Helen R. demonstrates the evil consequences of gossip, and a rigid and romantic code of moral conduct. This case is especially significant because it shows*

CHAPTER SEVEN

AUTHOR'S PREFACE

A NERVOUS breakdown is a terrifying experience. When it occurs, the patient, his family, and often his friends are panic-stricken. No one knows just what to do with the patient, and the patient is incapable of helping himself. Everyone offers gratuitous and conflicting advice. Sometimes the patient is stubbornly resistant to all good counsel. Often he tries everything in turn, only to become more confused and perplexed by the contradictory treatments to which he is exposed. Days of anxiety pass into weeks of mistrust, while the patient loses both his hope and his courage.

What should be done? If you think you have a nervous breakdown, it is your first duty to consult a competent and reputable physician, preferably your family doctor, and get a thorough and complete physical examination. If you cannot find any evidence of physical or organic disease, ask your doctor to recommend a reputable psychiatrist or medical psychologist. The psychiatrist is the physician whose training and experience best fits him to help you. To consult him is a sign of intelligence, not evidence of a weakened will or deranged mind.

Competent and sympathetic psychiatrists unfortunately are not always available. The burden of the nervous breakdown sometimes falls upon the family doctor, often upon the family and the friends of the patient, but eventually upon the patient himself, for it is he who must seek light and find guidance for his own salvation. This handbook is written, therefore, with a three-fold purpose: to guide the general practitioner in his treatment; to help the patient's family and friends to understand the patient's conduct and to avoid tragic errors in their counsel and aid; but, primarily, to help the patient to help himself.

You, who have a nervous breakdown, are the " forgotten man " of medicine. Few there are who can appreciate your anguish and your perplexity, fewer still who can assuage your inner conflict or console you in your grief. If you have already discovered that your nervous breakdown is at best a temporary palliative, if you have broken through to the profound psychological realisation that your breakdown, after months of doubt, conflict, and depression, does not work, I have written this book for you. Follow its counsel, and you will hasten the natural process of cure which you have already begun. You have nothing to fear. You can be helped. And I have written this book for you who have not yet learned this essential truth, in the hope that you will read beyond this preface, and, discovering the true meaning of the nervous breakdown, will be encouraged to find new and better methods of attaining peace and happiness. No matter how long you have had your nervous breakdown, it is not too late to learn how to be normal.

This is a compact manual of help and self-help. In

the first chapters I have explained just what a nervous breakdown is, what its usual causes are, and how its symptoms develop. Then I have traced the critical situations in which a nervous breakdown is likely to occur, how it works in these situations as a means of rescuing a crumbling sense of self-esteem, and why it fails to accomplish its purpose.

In the subsequent chapters I have described the more usual types of nervous breakdown, and have analysed in detail a complete case history illustrative of each type, so that you can sit behind the scenes and watch just how a nervous breakdown occurred, why it happened, and how that particular case was cured. To be sure, every nervous breakdown is unique. Your breakdown is unique. But there are certain general laws that apply to all breakdowns, and by reading these cases you will be able to discover these general laws and apply them to your own case.

In these chapters you will find cases of breakdown that occurred in adolescence and others that happened during university life. Then there are nervous breakdowns originating in various social situations. A variety of cases are presented in which the sexual problems are the basis of the breakdown. Cases due to an ignorance of the art and technique of love, cases based on the problem of masturbation, cases of nervous breakdown in women who were dissatisfied with being " just women ", and finally, cases dealing with the tragedies of romantic love and homosexuality are described in these chapters.

Then I have added an analysis of the vast number of nervous breakdowns which are based upon economic factors. Cases in which the loss of money or position are the critical factors are discussed in great detail, the causes of these distressing breakdowns are analysed, and practical suggestions made for recovery and rehabilitation. A section of the book is devoted to the breakdowns that arise directly from family conflicts. Cases of breakdown in middle age and in old age are analysed and described. You will see your own case mirrored in the stories of these men and women who have suffered a nervous breakdown, fought it out, and won.

The final chapters are packed with practical suggestions. These suggestions are not just theoretical counsels; they have passed the acid test of private and clinical practice. They have been tried in hundreds of cases and found to be successful. You will be amazed at their simplicity, and the ease with which they may be applied to your own case. They require nothing but a minimum of courage, of good will, and of imagination for their success. One warning: you will not find in this book any magical formula for cure. No nervous breakdown was ever cured without the patient's risking something. But the risk is really not great. A nervous breakdown is the most painful strategy of life, as anyone who has ever had one will attest. The good life, the normal life, on the other hand, is the easiest possible way to live. The cost of a nervous breakdown in suffering is out of all proportion to its dividends in security. A nervous breakdown may "save your face" in a critical situation, but its upkeep is ruinous and eventually it defeats its own ends. In these chapters you will learn a technique which will relieve you of the agonies of your nervous breakdown. It is my hope that you will not stop when you have arrived at this first goal, but will go on and become an artist in the art of creative self-realisation as well. I give you courage and the will to get well!

At this point, I wish to express my grateful appreciation to my secretary, Gertrude Silverman, for her valuable help in preparing this manuscript, and also to my patients, who, in sharing their troubles with me, have become my teachers and have given me insight and understanding of the dynamic processes of the nervous breakdown. I am especially indebted to those patients who have graciously consented to allow me to use their life stories, disguised to assure complete anonymity, as illustrative material for my book. If the recital of their perplexities, their training, and their final clarification will serve to encourage other sufferers to follow in their paths, their suffering will not have been in vain, and their cures more than a personal victory for them. I ask no greater recompense for the work of preparing this volume than that those who find insight and encouragement in these pages will, in turn, share their knowledge with some fellow man who has not yet learned how to be happy though human.

W. BÉRAN WOLFE.

CHAPTER ONE

OF CAUSES

What is a Nervous Breakdown?—How a Nervous Breakdown Originates—The Basic Laws of Human Nature—Fear and Ignorance: Fundamental Causes of Nervous Breakdown—The Critical Situations of Life—The Sense of "Face"—How We Maintain Our "Face"—Nervous Breakdown as a "Face-Saving" Device—How the Nervous Breakdown Works—Why the Nervous Breakdown Fails to Save "Face"—How a Nervous Breakdown is Cured—Looking Forward

EVERYONE knows what a knock-out is. A prize-fighter takes a terrific punch on the chin. He lies unconscious in the ring while the referee slowly counts him out. The prize-fighter has been so badly hurt that his body cannot function normally. Nature in her infinite wisdom has suspended his vital activities to keep him from killing himself. While the pugilist lies prostrate and insensible to the world about him, nature is carefully restoring his physical equilibrium. However ignominious the knock-out may be from the prize-fighter's personal point of view, it is a life-saving device so far as nature is concerned. The prize-fighter considers his knock-out as if it were a physical disaster. If he were only as wise as nature, he would understand that his knock-out is an emergency measure, designed to save him from the untoward results of his own physical folly.

A nervous breakdown may be described as a personality knock-out. In the arena of life we are sometimes exposed to sudden or intolerably severe shocks. In a physical knock-out the body alone gives up the struggle. In a nervous breakdown the whole personality declares a moratorium of normal activities, and both body and soul join in a cry for help. Both the knock-out and the nervous breakdown are merciful provisions of nature. The physical knock-out warns the prize-fighter that he has overstepped his physical powers of endurance. The nervous breakdown is a similar warning that you have broken the basic laws of human conduct.

When a prize-fighter is knocked out it denotes one of two things: either he does not know how to fight, or he has been matched against an opponent who is overwhelmingly superior. If you have a nervous breakdown it also signifies one of two things: you have not learned how to live, or you have suddenly been exposed to such overwhelming experiences that your personality has not been able to withstand the strain. Is a nervous breakdown a sign of weakness? Not at all. You have put up a good fight, but the odds were too heavy against you. Sometimes a weakling goes through life without ever having a breakdown, simply because he has never been subjected to a critical test. A strong man and an able fighter, on the other hand, may succumb to the onslaught of a gang of ruffians. Psychologically, the nervous breakdown indicates only one thing: your personality has been subjected to a strain too great for *you* to bear. Nature has warned you and given you respite. The breakdown is a definite indication that you are still functioning, and have within you the material for recovery.

HOW A NERVOUS BREAKDOWN ORIGINATES

We human beings have been living on this earth for some millions of years. Our animal ancestors preceded us by many more millions of years. The first living cell probably appeared on the earth billions of years ago. The cells that make up the human body are very similar to those primitive one-celled animals which were the ancestors of all living things. In the course of those billions of years of evolution from amoeba to man, the cells of our bodies have acquired a profound wisdom. We are not always aware of this primitive wisdom of our bodies. The sagacity of the cell lies outside our knowledge and consciousness, and if the cells of our bodies performed only the functions that we know they perform, in all probability we could not live more than a few minutes. We become conscious of this wisdom of the body only when we transgress the laws of normal living.

Consider, for example, the small boy who eats green apples. He unwittingly commits a sin against nature. It isn't a religious or moral sin, but a hygienic sin, a sin against the wisdom of the body. The wise old cells, tissues, and organs of his body broadcast a protest. We call that protest a stomach-ache. Although the stomach-ache is very annoying to the small boy, it is really a very favourable reaction on the part of his body. It shows that the cells of his stomach are on the job, protesting against the poison contained in green apples. If the small boy continued eating the green apples without being warned that he was committing a hygienic sin, he might eat himself into his grave. We sympathise with the youngster, but we are happy that he is the richer for this valuable experience.

In the course of these millions of years of evolution as human beings, we have not only acquired a certain physiological wisdom but also a psychological wisdom which is usually outside our conscious knowledge or understanding. Sometimes we commit psychological sins against our own humanity. We are ignorant of the fact that we are breaking a basic law of human nature when we commit these psychological sins, just as the small boy is completely ignorant of the fact that he is breaking a hygienic law when he eats the tempting green apples. The result is that we experience feelings of fear, depression, or anxiety. In the psychological sphere these anxiety feelings or depressions are comparable to the stomach-ache in the purely physiological sphere. They are the signals of warning, danger signs, that originate in the profoundest depths of our unconscious personalities.

In bygone ages it used to be believed that a human being was made up of two parts: his body and his soul. Modern science teaches us that this idea is no longer acceptable. We know that body and soul are just two different ways of looking at the same thing, the indestructible unity which we call the personality. We cannot divide the personality, although we can look at it from several points of view for the sake of convenience. Any human being is an indestructible unit moving toward a goal of security and happiness. You cannot divorce his body from his mind, his intellect from his emotions, his glands from his feelings, his bodily structure from his psychological conduct. Body and soul are simply different aspects of this same goal-seeking unity, the individual, the personality.

Thus it may happen that the small boy who eats the green apples may, under certain circumstances, suffer more from shame and remorse than from his stomach-ache, just as the mature business man, who somehow has run foul of the laws of human nature, may suffer from a headache or from sleeplessness, rather than from anxiety or depression. In some cases the cells of the body become the loudspeakers for the soul, and in other cases the reverse happens. It amounts to this: you break one of the laws of hygiene. Nature will give you a warning signal. The signal may come from the body, or it may come from the mind. Sometimes it comes from both simultaneously. If you stop transgressing the natural law, the signal will stop. If you do not stop, the signal will become more intense. If you persist despite nature's warnings, nature will knock you out. A nervous breakdown is a psychological knock-out.

You have a nervous breakdown. I wish there were a better word to describe it, because a nervous breakdown is not really a breakdown, and it has practically nothing to do with your nerves. Let us say, for the time being, that you have declared a personality moratorium. As soon as you recognize this important fact you are immediately in possession of ten important sets of facts: 1. You have transgressed the laws of nature, but you have put up a good fight, attempting to have the last word. Nature has given you a personality knock-out to save you from the consequences of your own folly. This does not mean you are a weakling. It means simply that no man can pit his private opinion against nature and win. 2. Nature has given you a warning signal that you may no longer disregard. 3. The damage is not too great to repair. If it were, you would not be reading this book. 4. There is some mistake in your strategy of life which has brought you into conflict with nature and reality. 5. The warning signal which nature has given you may be annoying, but you should be happy that you have perceived it. The sooner you learn you are on the wrong road, the quicker and the easier your recovery will be. 6. In the face of the overwhelming evidence of a mistaken strategy of life, the sensible thing to do is to examine the pattern of your life and discover just what mistakes you have made. 7. The less time you waste complaining about your symptoms or indulging in orgies of self-pity, the better. Every minute spent in complaining delays your cure just so much. 8. It is folly to try your old strategy of life all over again. A nervous breakdown is a sign of a *basic* mistake. If you do the same thing all over again, but try to do it more intensely, you will get another personality knock-out for your pains. You cannot beat nature. 9. As soon as you have learned where you have made your mistakes, begin training *consciously* toward a normal goal. Your symptoms will disappear as if by magic as soon as you have begun the work of personality reconstruction. 10. You are not too old nor too weak to begin over again. Much of what you have learned in the course of your life is still useful, although you have abused that knowledge in the past by applying it to false ends. The fact that you have a nervous breakdown indicates that you have ample powers of resistance. It isn't too late to be normal.

THE BASIC LAWS OF HUMAN NATURE

What are the basic facts of human nature that you must take into consideration in planning for happiness, security, and a sense of well-being? Here you are on a crust of earth, subjected to certain atmospheric, climatic, chemical, biological, historical, economic, and social conditions. The following laws of human nature have proved themselves to be fairly constant and unchanging. The future may add new laws or subtract from the old ones. You are living in the present and for the present they will give you a good working philosophy of conduct. Incorporate these laws into your life and you will not make any tragic mistakes.

1. Human beings must work or starve. If they do not have to work to live, they must busy themselves to keep from dying of sheer boredom.

2. No human being is alone in the world. His conduct, therefore, must always take the welfare of his fellow men into consideration. If a man is interested only in himself, and he isolates himself from his fellow men, he not only transgresses a basic law of human nature, but denies himself all opportunities of attaining personal significance. All human values are basically social values.

3. Human beings are divided into two sexes to facilitate the propagation of the race. If a human being is not interested in members of the opposite sex, the sexual equilibrium of nature is disturbed. It is folly to deny one's sexuality.

4. Human beings are endowed with minds in order to help them solve the foregoing complicated problems of work, leisure, society and sex. The solution of these problems is a full-time job for the normal mind. To divert the human mind from the solution of these real problems, and to occupy it with metaphysical or occult problems, is one way to prepare for a nervous breakdown.

5. The human infant is the weakest creature in the world.

6. The mind of the child develops faster than his body. The human infant is unique among all living things in this one respect: he is the only living thing that *experiences* a sense of his own inadequacy. The

young of other animals are weak. The human child *knows* he is weak, long before he can do anything about it.

7. While the feeling of inferiority is a universal experience for all human beings, no human being can bear to *remain* inferior. All human beings strive to grow, to become strong, superior and secure.

8. The pattern of any individual's life is a pattern of compensation for the inferiority feeling experienced in childhood. Nature has endowed us richly with compensatory mechanisms, both physical and psychological. The strategy of any individual's life is directed toward a goal of security, superiority, and well-being. Human happiness consists in the *perception of progress* toward this goal.

9. The individual human goal of security and happiness is an *unconscious* goal. It is fixed in our unconscious minds in early childhood, long before the development of our mature critical faculties, and, therefore, it often lies beyond the bounds of human attainment. To strive for an unattainable goal, a goal of godlikeness, a goal of superhuman attainment, is to court a personality disaster.

10. The attainment of security, well-being, superiority, and human happiness, is the goal of life. Happiness, however, is not an object, and cannot be pursued as an object. Happiness is an attribute of the good life. The good life consists in the conscious mobilisation of your faculties and talents for the attainment of a conscious goal of compensation. This goal must

lie within the boundaries of human attainment, and must encompass the correct solution of the problems of work, leisure, sex and society. To attempt less than this goal is to remain a victim of an intolerable sense of inferiority. To attempt more is to transgress the laws of reality, and to risk a personality disaster.

If you analyse these ten laws of human nature you will see that there are really two sets of facts contained in them. The first set applies to mankind in general, and has to do with the maintenance of the human race. The second set applies to you, as an individual, and the laws of your personal development. Society expects you to become a contributing, co-operative member. You, of course, have private goals and ends, because you are human, and because you once felt the inferiority of being a child in a grown-up world. Your chief personal goal is to transform the "minus" situation of your childhood into a "plus" situation of security, satisfaction and self-esteem. The best and perhaps the only way to do this is to arrange your life in such a way that your pattern of compensation shall simultaneously contribute to the happiness and security of the social group in which you live.

FEAR AND IGNORANCE: FUNDMENTAL CAUSES OF NERVOUS BREAKDOWN

There are a great many unhappy people in the world. Most of their unhappiness is quite unnecessary. Much of the avoidable unhappiness of human beings, as you may have surmised, originates in the conflict between the individual's desire for personal superiority and society's demand that each individual conform to and co-operate in the social task. Analyse an unhappy life, and you will usually find that the unhappy man has either set his goal of security and satisfaction beyond the pale of human attainment, or beyond the bounds of social approval. The unhappy man is haunted by a persistent sense of inferiority which he has failed to compensate in a socially approved fashion. Because of this persistent inferiority complex he refuses to be "just another average man". He wants to play the part of God, and therein lies the fundamental basis of his unhappiness. But the desire to play God is essentially no more than ignorance of the delights of being human, and fear of the responsibilities of social co-operation.

Ignorance is the mother of fear; fear in turn breeds egoism, isolation, and abnormal demands for security and personal superiority. Egoism, isolation and illogical desires for the guarantee of complete security, in their turn, lead to unsocial conduct. A certain amount of egoism, isolation and lack of social co-operation is tolerated by society at large. Beyond that limit conflicts between the egoist and society are unavoidable. It is just at this point of unavoidable conflict that the nervous breakdown occurs in the struggling egoist, who feels that adjustment to the laws of social co-operation is beyond his power.

In this brief history of the nervous breakdown I cannot describe in detail the many origins of fear and ignorance. The most usual of these are physical or organic handicaps, competition with brothers or sisters, the widespread struggle for domination between the sexes, the social, economic, religious, or racial situations in which the individual finds himself in a hated minority group, and especially the unfavourable emotional influence of parents and teachers. Sometimes it is the parents' hate, neglect, undue authority, or nagging that does the damage to the child. The "great expectations" of parents, their vanity, and particularly their pampering, coddling, and over-solicitous protection of their children, are all capable of fostering the child's inferiority feelings. These untoward parental attitudes lay the basis for a life of dependence, isolation, uncooperativeness, conflict, and unhappiness. *The indispensable pre-requisites of a happy life are courage, social co-operation, and spiritual independence.* Any factors in the life of the child which damage the development of these qualities almost inevitably lead to discouragement, hopelessness, and an uncontrolled striving for personal superiority. Thus is laid the basis for a future nervous breakdown.[1]

[1] The reader is referred to the author's *How to be Happy Though Human* (Routledge, 1932) for a more complete description of the inferiority complex, its origins, manifestations, and false compensations.

THE CRITICAL SITUATIONS OF LIFE

If we are correct in our analysis of the causes of the nervous breakdown, it would follow logically that a nervous breakdown might be expected to occur at a period of greater strain, or in some critical situation in which courage, social co-operation, independence, and a well-developed sense of self-esteem were indispensable requisites of success. Clinical evidence supports this logical conclusion. No nervous breakdown is an accident. In many of the cases of complete nervous breakdown that occur in maturity, moreover, we discover a history of minor breakdowns in the previous crises of the patient's childhood, adolescence, and early adult life. Had these minor breakdowns been understood and correctly interpreted, the proper training for normality might have been instituted, and the subsequent breakdowns forestalled or entirely prevented. The case histories of men and women who suffer from nervous breakdown indicate that almost every nervous breakdown has some antecedent history of premonitory anxieties and failures. And there is every evidence to indicate that, almost without exception, nervous breakdowns occur most frequently in certain typical "critical" situations. These are the dangerous corners on the highroad of life.

Life becomes critical to some individuals in the very first days of existence. A child is born with organic defects that immediately unfit it for the world. Sometimes the critical situation lies in the mistaken emotional attitudes of "illegitimate" parents. An unwanted child is actually born into a critical situation. An almost universal critical situation develops when a child is weaned from its mother's breast and compelled to eat independently. Early childhood is replete with difficulties. Sleeping alone, eating alone, the conquest of the dark, learning to walk and to talk, may all be critical situations for the child. Among the more common of these dangerous corners of childhood is the birth of a younger brother or sister. Nothing can be so tragic in the child's life as the experience of being dethroned by a weak and unwelcome little usurper of its mother's love. This is one of the reasons we find so many nervous breakdowns in eldest children. Severe illness, or the death of a parent, is also frequently the signal for the appearance of a childhood breakdown.

We do not call the behaviour of a child who has temper tantrums when she has been weaned a true nervous breakdown, but, psychologically, it is equivalent to this same child's fit of hysterics twenty-five years later when the problems of marriage threaten her security in the immediate future. A nervous breakdown is rarely an isolated phenomenon. It is the product of a long process of unconscious training that has usually begun before the child's sixth year of age. The battle of Waterloo, so the historians claim, was won on the playing fields of Eton. But it is much more certain that the defeats of adult life are rooted in the tragedies of the nursery, in the frustrations of the breakfast table, and in the failures experienced on the playground and in the kindergarten.

Perhaps the commonest critical situation of childhood is the experience of going to school. In the school, that testing ground of the early childhood training for social co-operation, we have a true epitome of the larger battlefields of life. The so-called "problem" behaviour of young school children is the equivalent of the neurosis of the adult. If every school were equipped with a properly organised and directed psychological child guidance clinic, the nervous breakdowns of adult life would be reduced to a minimum, because the prevention of mental breakdowns is more successfully accomplished by the child guidance clinic than by any other institution. During the school period the critical situations of puberty are often superimposed on the social and occupational adjustments of earlier school days. For many girls, the beginning of menstruation; for many boys, the changing of the voice, the first growth of the beard, and the appearance of secondary sexual characteristics, mark the end of a happy childhood and the beginning of the first frustrations of mature life.

After school, critical situations come thick and fast. For many young men the transition from the protective atmosphere of school or university to the harsher competition of the business and social world is in itself a critical test of the personality. Entrance into the world of economic competition is one of the commonest critical situations. Sexual maturity and the necessity of making an adequate adjustment to members of the opposite sex; marriage, pregnancy, childbirth, fatherhood—all of these are critical situations.

In middle-age economic insecurity, or the prospect of a loss of sexual virility, is frequently the occasion for a nervous breakdown. Leisure may become a critical problem at this time. The necessity of meeting old difficulties with lessened physical vigour and ability may signalise the onset of a breakdown.

In this period the recognition of the hopelessness of childhood ambitions is also likely to occur. Children who "go wrong" or fail to come up to their parents' expectations may be the occasion of a personality disaster in their parents. The prospect of dependence, the fear of growing old, and the ever present fear of death are other critical situations that often cause a spiritual declaration of bankruptcy. At all times, the loss of a mate or child or a long-held position, economic reverses, social tragedies, scandal, or severe disease may produce that sense of futility and unreality which is the forerunner of every nervous breakdown.

THE SENSE OF "FACE"

Before we proceed with the description of the nervous breakdown we must say something about the concept of "face" which is essential to the understanding of the nervous breakdown. We, of the Western world, like to believe that the Orientals have developed this idea of "face" to an exaggerated degree. This is not true. Ideas and ideals of "face" vary with time and geography, but every living man and woman has a certain irreducible minimum standard of self-esteem, without which life is not worth living. A high police official may not commit suicide by disembowelling himself because a murder remains unsolved during his tenure of office, but he might easily have a nervous breakdown if he found himself penniless after gambling on the Stock Exchange, or if some enterprising newspaper reporter published a too lurid *exposé* of police scandal during his administration. The Occidental sense of "face" is less dramatic than the Oriental, and manifests itself in different forms, but it is just as real. It is as if every human being walked through life holding a mask in front of his face. This mask is a double mask. One side represents the you that *you* would like to be. The other side represents the you that you want the *world* to know you as. The mask serves two purposes. It keeps you from having a bad opinion of yourself, and it keeps the world from discovering how inferior you really know yourself to be.

"Face" is an essential of life. The reason we spend our lives "saving our face" is that no man dares look at himself as he really is. The aspect would be too humiliating and too devastating. Nature, whose only purpose is the maintenance of the race, has given us the creative ability to fashion a romantic camouflage about our personalities, to the end that we may continue to perform the task of living. Without "face" life becomes intolerable. Without an intact sense of "face" no man can tackle the objective problems of reality; without "face" we are not human.

The maintenance of "face" is the essential unconscious occupation of every human being. The normal, objective, courageous, independent, happy, well-adjusted human being bases his sense of "face" on his usefulness to his fellow men. The neurotic individual constructs his sense of self-esteem on untenable and uncertain foundations. It is apparent that if you think you are worthless unless you have a million in the bank, you not only do not think much of yourself, but also you are haunted by the fear that you may at any moment be reduced to a sense of intolerable inferiority by factors entirely beyond your control. If you base your sense of self-esteem or "face" on purely subjective, fictional, neurotic, or otherwise untenable premises, your whole life becomes one long critical situation, and at any moment it may become necessary for you to have a nervous breakdown to save it. Human happiness is impossible unless you construct your sense of " face " upon the certain foundations of the basic laws of human nature.

HOW WE MAINTAIN OUR " FACE "

If you were to investigate the flimsy supports on which neurotic individuals construct their sense of " face ", you would not be astonished at the number of nervous breakdowns that occur. One of my patients had a nervous breakdown because a pimple appeared on her cheek. For eighteen years she had based her self-esteem solely on her flawless complexion! Another patient suffered a complete nervous prostration because he failed in his first year's examination in mathematics. As might be expected, his father was a well-known university professor of mathematics and had coached his son to be a second Einstein.

The sense of " face " is as varied as the shape of the human nose. " Face " may be based on physical beauty, muscular prowess, or simply animal health. It may be constructed on the indispensable love or approval of a parent, brother, wife, husband, grandfather, or child. I have seen a man feeling blue and depressed because his favourite dog ran after a stranger (who probably had a ham sandwich in his pocket) instead of answering to his master's call.

"Face" may be based on any superiority, real or fancied, whether it be the ability to decipher Egyptian hieroglyphics or virtuosity in mixing cocktails. It may be based on intellectual development and it may depend on stupidity, as in the case of the schoolboy who based his self-esteem on the fact that he was the only boy in his class who couldn't be taught the multiplication table. "Face" is often founded in the possession of chattels, whether these be money, postage stamps, old masters, or gilt-edge securities. It may be constructed on any technical virtuosity, from the ability to play a Chopin waltz in two minutes and thirty-six seconds, to flag-pole sitting, marathon dancing, sexual conquests, or the ability to train fleas.

To many people "face" connotes the ability to be the first, the best, the tallest, the wisest, the most macabre, the meanest, the oldest or the youngest this or that. To others, "face" consists solely in some form of subjective and futile uniqueness. Power, in whatever form, is an essential ingredient of the sense of "face". Whatever its basis, and no matter how bizarre its form, every man's sense of "face" must connote a superiority, an individual and personal virtuosity which satisfies and compensates him for other inadmissible or unconfessed inferiorities. In a word "face" is the crystallisation, in some specific form, of the individual's striving for godlike superiority.

Whatever the form or substance of the sense of

" face ", its maintenance is an essential of all human happiness. *A sense of " face " based on service to one's fellow men is the only secure basis of self-esteem, because it is the only one that permits constant and conscious control.* This basis alone takes into consideration the fundamental facts of social organisation, gives proper expression to the creative power in every human being, and is independent of external conditions. Money may be lost, sexual virility may wane, beauty may fade, and health may give way to sickness; youth may turn to old age and even great intellect may degenerate into querulous pedantry. A sense of " face " based on the possession of any of these is insecure. A sense of " face " constructed only on such transient foundations compels you to spend most of your life protecting your self-esteem from the onslaughts of the world of reality. The more varied your service and usefulness to your fellow men is, the more certain you are that your sense of self-esteem is secure. The vast majority of men and women, nevertheless, persists in putting all its eggs into one basket despite the antiquity of the advice against such conduct. When some single and inadequate container of your precious self-esteem is destroyed, you are confronted with the disaster of a loss of " face ". The panic and perplexity which follow a loss of " face " we call " nervous breakdown ".

During and after the Russian Revolution countless men and women suffered such nervous breakdowns, because their only basis of self-esteem was their claim to genealogical nobility. After the American Civil War, numberless freed slaves returned voluntarily to slavery, because their childish sense of " face " depended solely on their irresponsible attachment to their former masters. They simply could not conceive of themselves as personally responsible for their happiness. In the present economic collapse, thousands of people, and especially Americans, have suffered nervous breakdowns because they had mistakenly based their self-esteem entirely upon the fatness of their bank accounts. The fiction that " money is power " had indeed become so widespread in the United States that the deflation of American paper prosperity produced a veritable national hysteria, tragically comparable to the tears and lamentations of a child who has discovered that there is no Santa Claus.

NERVOUS BREAKDOWN AS A " FACE-SAVING " DEVICE

We must make the relation between the loss of " face " and the occurrence of a nervous breakdown absolutely clear. As we have said, the maintenance of " face " is the one basic profession of every man, woman and child. To lose " face " is to admit an intolerable worthlessness. We must maintain our masks at all costs. Sometimes a nervous breakdown *follows* a loss of " face ", and very frequently it *precedes* the personality crisis. *The nervous break-*

down, then, is not a weakness, but is a valuable unconscious offensive-defensive device designed to save " face " before personality disaster occurs. How does the nervous breakdown " save face "? In a variety of ways, depending on the individual, his physical and intellectual constitution, his environment, and the nature of the supports which he has fashioned for his sense of " face ". In another chapter we shall explain in detail why the nervous breakdown is an ineffectual " face-saving " device. At this point we wish only to demonstrate how the nervous breakdown accomplishes its unconscious purpose.

HOW THE NERVOUS BREAKDOWN WORKS

In some cases, as we have said, the nervous breakdown occurs during a critical situation but *before* the sense of " face " actually has been assaulted. It is comparable to an army's " digging in " for a long siege. In these cases the nervous breakdown can be interpreted as a plea for exoneration, for exculpation, for leniency, or for " extenuating circumstances ". It is as if the individual with the nervous breakdown were saying: " Look at me! I am a sick man. You cannot expect anything of me! " The reader must understand that *this nervous breakdown is in no sense a conscious evasion of the responsibilities of the critical situation.* It is either completely or partially an *unconscious* phenomenon. If you give up in the face of a difficulty or responsibility, which often seems quite an ordinary duty to your neighbours, you lay yourself open to the charge of being a slacker. This indictment would be just as intolerable to your sense of " face " as if you had actually failed. The man with the nervous breakdown has no *insight* into the connection between his symptoms and the problem he is evading. In order to deceive others he must first delude himself.

When you have a nervous breakdown, you look to the past for an explanation of your present symptoms, expecting that the law of cause and effect, which governs so many natural phenomena, will also explain these strange sensations. But the meaning of your breakdown is not to be found in the past, except in so far as the past will reveal the existence of factors of discouragement which play a rôle in your present threatened loss of " face ". *The real meaning and significance of a nervous breakdown must be sought in the future.* Thus, a man has a nervous breakdown on the eve of his marriage. He attributes his symptoms to overwork in his profession. Ask him what he would do if he were cured in twenty-four hours, and he would immediately answer, " I'd get married and go on my honeymoon! " Now his breakdown unmasks itself as an *unconscious evasion* of a new responsibility in a critical situation. He lacks confidence in his ability to carry out the obligations of marriage. Society demands that he tackle the new responsibilities. To fail would be to lose " face ". The nervous breakdown, on the specious plea of overwork (which he may unconsciously have driven himself to do in order to bolster his excuse with objective data), is thus an offensive- (against marriage) defensive (" face-saving ") device in which body and soul work harmoniously for the preservation of the integrity of his ego.

In other cases the nervous breakdown occurs *after* the " face " mask has been suddenly destroyed or violently displaced. This type of breakdown occurs frequently in individuals who have based their existence upon the support of some one human being, whose affection or help has become an indispensable condition of their continued activity. We call such a relation a psychological symbiosis. There are many examples of dependent relationship—symbiosis—in nature. The best one is the lichen, which is not one plant but two plants, a moss and an alga, living as one. Another example is the relation between the flower and the bee. The flower allows the bee to take its honey but benefits by the fact that the bee, in turn, helps to carry its pollen to another flower. Psychological symbiosis is not at all uncommon in human relations.

When a psychological symbiotic relationship between two people is dissolved by the death, removal, or unwillingness of the " host " to maintain the relationship, the *dependent* member of the psychological symbiosis often has a nervous breakdown. Such a nervous breadown is equivalent to a frantic cry for help. Here the breakdown is again an offensive-defensive strategy. It launches an offensive against the unwilling "host", as if the dependent individual were saying: "See what you have done to me! How you have made me suffer! How heartless you are! You must come back and re-establish the relation!" The defensive aspect lies in the individual's unconscious justification to himself: "If I were not so sick I would now become an independent and self-reliant individual. But see how helpless and incapable I really am! No one can expect anything of me in this situation!"

There is a vast difference in the natural grief of a self-reliant individual who has lost a loved one, and the frantic lamentations of the dependent member of a psychological symbiosis who has lost his host, just as there is a vast difference between the sudden shock and chagrin of a normal individual who sees the fruit of a life's work snatched from him by circumstances beyond human control, and the petulant rage of a spoiled child who has been denied his customary lollypop. It is the difference between grief and bathos, between shock and hysterics. The individual with the nervous breakdown frequently overplays his part in his anxiety to effect his unconscious purpose. His pains are always "terrible", "frightful", "incredible", his suffering always "unbearable torture", his anguish dramatically "heart-rending". To the trained observer his grief and anguish seem unreal, the " uniqueness " of his situation approaches the supernatural. The psychologically trained physician looks for a critical situation when the patient enters his consulting room with the avowal, " Doctor, I'm sure you've never seen a case like mine." And yet, if you have ever had a nervous breakdown, you know how real, how agonising, how intolerable these symptoms are. And that brings us to the next point, the ineffectuality of the nervous breakdown.

WHY THE NERVOUS BREAKDOWN FAILS TO SAVE "FACE"

If the nervous breakdown is such an excellent device for saving " face ", and if " face " must be saved, why should we attempt to *cure* a nervous breakdown? There may be a few occasions when a breakdown of the personality compels the individual to cease from too arduous labours, but these are rare cases. Usually the nervous breakdown is an ineffectual method of saving one's " face " although it appears at first glance as the method of choice. In the vast majority of cases in which the nervous breakdown occurs, the sense of " face " is based on artificial and unsound values beyond human realisation. In these same cases we find that the breakdown is based on an unwarranted fear of reality, the roots of which are to be found in the discouraged ignorance of childhood experiences. In other words, a nervous breakdown is too high a price to pay for the upkeep of a sense of " face " which is socially sick and not worth saving.

In the examination of a case of nervous breakdown we are frequently struck with the patient's over-emphasis of symptoms. The pain, as we have already mentioned, is always " intolerable ", the anguish " incredible ". This over-emphasis of the *uniqueness* of the symptoms—which is absolutely real and tangible to the patient, and not " put on " as some physicians and relatives are inclined to believe—leads us to the conclusion of Hamlet's mother: " The lady doth protest too much methinks." Perhaps the victim of the nervous breakdown does vaguely realise that his symptoms have an air of unreality, and he compels himself to make them more vivid. When we find that a patient must undergo prolonged sieges of self-torment, self-torture, self-sabotage, remorse, shame, and humiliation, we can hardly fail to agree with him that a nervous breakdown is not worth the candle.

When you have a nervous breakdown, your fear of meeting the responsibilities of adult life is further aggravated by the fear that your symptoms will be discovered and unmasked as an escape from responsibility. Every friend and every member of your family becomes a potential detective who may disclose your unconscious guilt. This compels you to isolate yourself further, and so adds additional discouragement to your despair. Isolation leads to reduplication and intensification of your symptoms.

You become inextricably involved in rationalisations, evasions, and further flights from objective reality. Finally you become confused by the very virtuosity of your symptoms, and the more you attempt to rid yourself of their torture, the deeper you sink into chaotic panic.

The timid individual who is faced with an obstacle that threatens a personality disaster, quails at the thought of irrevocable defeat, and saves his " face " by the unconscious construction and arrangement of the breakdown. The purpose of this breakdown is the avoidance of the responsibility that must be born in facing the critical situation. The arrangement of the symptoms transforms his " I am afraid to try lest I be defeated " into " I cannot, because my sickness prevents me, although I really have the best of intentions to meet this challenge."

If you have a nervous breakdown you are completely hypnotised by the difficulties that lie in your path. Your breakdown seems a splendid way out. And so it would be, *were it not for the fact that the nervous breakdown involves greater emotional responsibilities than the responsibilities entailed by the objective problems that the breakdown is designed to avoid.* Once you have chosen the nervous breakdown as a way out, you have to nurture and train it. Perhaps you have already realised that your breakdown is a tyrannical Frankenstein. You are like the magician with a charm that is supposed to convey great powers. The charm turns against the wizard and drives him from his own home. A nervous breakdown requires absolute service and devotion as the price of protection. The drudgery of keeping up a nervous breakdown is a full-time job.

When you unconsciously choose a nervous breakdown as a way out of your difficulties, you eventually become the slave of your method instead of its master. Sooner or later, you, who have unconsciously arranged a nervous breakdown for the purpose of saving your " face ", will find that its costs in symptoms are out of all proportion to its dividends in security. Your remedy is worse than your ailment. You find yourself in the situation of the explorer who was travelling by canoe up the Amazon river. His craft struck a hidden reef, and in a brief moment all his equipment went swirling down within the current. In mortal fear of his life he swam out to what seemed to be a solid log jutting out from the shore, only to find to his horror, as he grasped what had seemed to be a life-saving spar, that he had embraced—a sleeping crocodile! The nervous breakdown does not work as a " face-saving " device. And even if it did work, its costs would still be out of all proportion to its benefits. That is why a nervous breakdown should be cured.

HOW A NERVOUS BREAKDOWN IS CURED

In a limited manual of this kind I cannot, unfortunately, go into great details about the treatment of a nervous breakdown. The reader must be content with the bare skeleton of my interpretation of the symptomatology of the nervous breakdown, and the briefest of indications concerning the dynamics of the cure. The patient who goes to a dentist with an aching tooth does all that he can to help the dentist to cure him. The patient with a nervous breakdown, however, often interposes every conceivable obstacle to his psychiatrist. Part of the technique of having a nervous breakdown consists in carefully deluding not only your family but also the psychologist whom you consult, and in leading him down the blind alley of philosophical discussion, or into other blind alleys of emotional resistance or over-attachment. The discussion of these dynamics would not be appropriate in a text for laymen. What we can do, however, is to analyse the steps that occur in the cure of any nervous breakdown.

No cure of a nervous breakdown is possible unless the patient retains enough insight to know that something is wrong with him. The *first* step in the cure, therefore, is the realisation that something is wrong. *The patient who comes to the realisation of the ineffectuality of his life's pattern spontaneously, and voluntarily consults a medical psychologist for help,* has already won more than half the battle. The *second* step in the cure is the realisation on the part of the patient with the nervous breakdown, that he cannot cure himself without some outside aid. This aid may come from a friend, a book, or from a psychologist, but it must come from the outside. If the patient *could* understand the purpose and meaning of his symptoms without outside help, *he would, spontaneously, have chosen a better way to live.* The reason that he has a nervous breakdown is that he has misinterpreted a present or future danger in terms of a faulty past experience. A clam knows the inside of his shell better than anyone else in the world, but his clamshell is a very small world. It requires someone with a different point of view to tell the clam whether he is secure in the sand or insecure in the clam-digger's bucket. The *third* step is the recognition of the whole galaxy of symptoms and the objective interpretation of their meaning.

Many victims of a nervous breakdown cause themselves untold pain because they have a romantic belief that they can " work it out for themselves ". While an occasional sufferer, by virtue of an apparent inspiration, the source of which he cannot trace, comes to the realisation of a new set of values and cures himself, such cases are rare. The cases of nervous breakdown that are cured spontaneously are usually " cured " because the critical situation becomes less threatening with time, or because someone comes to the sufferer's aid and lifts him bodily out of it. In such cases no true cure is effected because the sufferer has not gained any insight from his experience. He has simply laid himself open to future difficulties. Nothing could be more futile than the false pride of the patient who has a nervous breakdown. He is afraid of going to a psychiatrist because of the fallacious belief that psychiatrists treat only the insane. The modern psychiatrist is much more interested in the prevention of insanity than in its treatment.

If you are very timid about talking with a psychiatrist, or are very anxious that your friends and family remain ignorant of the fact that you are seeking help, a conversation with your physician will assure you that not only your confidences, but the very fact that you are seeking aid, will remain an absolute secret. Psychiatrists are human beings. They are best fitted by training to understand the problems of the nervous breakdown. To consult a psychiatrist, where a reputable psychiatrist is available, is a sign of intelligent insight into the nature of your problems. If you do not know whom to consult, ask your family doctor to call a reputable psychiatrist in consultation. And beware of self-styled "practical" psychologists, "mind-healers" and the like. A nervous breakdown is too serious a matter to leave to the tender mercies of an insufficiently trained layman.

The cure of the nervous breakdown, therefore,

consists of the following stages: (1) the patient knows something is wrong; (2) he recognises that he cannot understand the meaning and purpose of his breakdown without the objective collaboration of a properly trained psychiatrist; (3) he has the intelligence and the courage to seek aid. The next step, (4), is the study and understanding of the symptoms, (the critical situation, and the environment in which the nervous breakdown occurs), with the collaboration of the psychiatrist; and then, (5), the attainment of insight into the dynamics of the workings of the whole symptom-complex—that is, how the offensive-defensive strategy of the unconscious accomplishes its hidden purpose.

When this new insight is gained by the patient, the psychiatrist proceeds (6) to the examination of the patient's past life, the establishment of his pattern of life, and his unconscious goal in living. This includes the discussion of mistaken interpretations of critical situations in the past, of fallacious emotional patterns and attitudes. The patient, at this point, ought to understand why he has made his failures, and why he cannot go on making them without critical damage to himself. Some patients get well spontaneously when this understanding is reached. The new insight liberates them from the chains of past experiences, and mobilises their existing forces for the new life of normality. But in most cases further clarification is necessary.

In the next stage (7), the patient must be given a

new, objective, normal, and attainable goal in life. When this goal is set in accordance with the circumstances and environment of the patient, a new training, (8), (as above) must be begun toward the normal goal. At this point many individuals come to the first realisation of their false patterns, and shrink back from the new critical situation that is caused by their insight and the necessity of doing something about it. The old symptoms that vanished in the first few conferences with the psychiatrist are likely to recur, and occasionally in more aggravated form. This should never be taken as a sign of a relapse. It is rather an indication that the patient has come to a higher level of insight, and is protesting (with his old symptoms) that he cannot go on. The recurrence of old symptoms at this time points to the fact that the psychiatrist has hit the bull's-eye. The patient sees himself in his true colours, and attempts to save " face " according to his old patterns.

When this occurs, (9), the psychiatrist must retrace the same ground again, encourage the patient, clarify the problems and help him by easy stages to build up his sense of " face " on solid ground. Here it is that our counsel (that symptoms are not arguments) must be taken by the patient more seriously than ever. The patient is in transition between his old neurotic pattern of life and a new, still mysterious, pattern of normality. The psychiatrist in a sense has given him a bad conscience. The patient realises that he cannot go back to his old symptoms, because he understands their meaning. He has not yet the courage to begin his new life. The psychiatrist requires a vast store of imagination, patience, and good will to help the sufferer over this last hurdle. He must unmask each new, unconscious trick that the patient develops in order to escape from the toils of objective reality. But as each symptom is put aside, the patient realises that there is one sympathetic human being who understands him, and this realisation helps him on his path.

Finally, (10), there comes that amazing clarification in which the patient suddenly sees himself in a new light: he has become a responsible human being who guides his destinies according to his *conscious* understanding of the problems of human happiness. He is no longer an irresponsible victim of circumstances. The erstwhile patient becomes the captain of a ship, steering its course to a known port, according to scientific charts and calculations. He is no longer a shipwrecked mariner, tossing on an ocean of unknown terrors in a rudderless and damaged life-boat, flying a hopeless signal of distress, drifting with the currents of fear, and being blown by the gales of ignorance where chance directs. And when you can say that insight and clarification have been translated into new and satisfying patterns of conduct, you can say truthfully, "I have cured myself of my nervous breakdown."

LOOKING FORWARD

The nervous breakdown is never quite as serious as it seems. It is, as we have already stated, a favourable symptom of a curable condition. Being based on fear, ignorance, an unstable and untenable sense of " face ", *the nervous breakdown can be cured by encouragement, knowledge and the extension of the foundations of the personality to the solid granite of objective activity in social co-operation.* The personality of the individual with a nervous breakdown is like a top spinning dizzily on the point of egoism. It is in unstable equilibrium because its centre of gravity lies outside its base of support, that is, outside the facts of social co-operation. The normal personality is like a pyramid, equipoised on four corner-stones: courage, independence, co-operation and common sense. It is easier to be a pyramid than a spinning top. If you have a nervous breakdown take Nature's warning for what it is worth. In the following pages you will find an explanation of your case and some practical, common-sense exercises in independence and social co-operation, to help you cure yourself. I give you courage and hope.

CHAPTER TWO

OF SYMPTOMS

The Galaxy of Symptoms—The Decalogue of the Nervous Breakdown—The Body Speaks: "Organ Jargon"—Emotional Symptoms in Nervous Breakdown—How the Symptoms Are Chosen—The Rôle of Complexes—How the Complex Works—Unconscious Strategies in Nervous Breakdown—Self-sabotage—Suicide and the Suicidal Impulse—Is Suicide Justifiable?—L'Envoi: Symptoms Are Not Arguments

THE GALAXY OF SYMPTOMS

IN THE foregoing chapter we discovered that the nervous breakdown, far from being a mysterious ailment of the nervous system, is in reality an offensive-defensive strategy of the total personality, exquisitely designed to save "face". We have found that the nervous breakdown is most likely to occur in certain critical situations in which the normal strains and stresses of life are exaggerated, and we have seen, moreover, that the breakdown is the result of a false strategy of life based on ignorance of certain fundamental laws of human nature, biology, and sociology. Our examination of the nervous breakdown has given us a new insight into the nature of its symptoms. We have discovered that the symptoms of the nervous breakdown, far from being evidence of weakness, represent healthy warnings (emanating from the immemorial wisdom of the body cells and tissues), which are subsequently elaborated by the total personality into a cry for help or leniency.

If you consider the complexity of human experience, the countless variations of the human body, and the unpredictable stresses of modern life, you will not be surprised to find that the symptoms of nervous breakdown are themselves almost infinite in their variety. To describe them in detail would require an encyclopedia, and would serve only to confuse you, especially if you have already been confused by your own symptoms or the cheerless dictum of your physician, "I can find nothing organically wrong with you!" In this chapter we shall discuss *types of symptoms* rather than symptoms themselves, so that you may understand their meaning in the *gestalt*, or total situation, of the sufferer. To begin with, you must realise three truths about the symptoms of the nervous breakdown: 1, all symptoms are relative; 2, each breakdown is different and unique in its form and manifestations; and 3, all breakdowns follow certain easily distinguishable patterns.

The first thing to remember about the symptoms of a nervous breakdown is that, since the breakdown is in itself a purposive, dynamic pattern of conduct, an unconscious strategy of life with a very definite goal, all the symptoms of the nervous breakdown must subserve the same purpose as the breakdown of which they are a part. The patient is not aware of this unconscious purpose, and has no *insight* into the nature of his symptoms. As we have said, the breakdown could not attain its purpose if the patient enjoyed his symptoms. In order that the breakdown should accomplish its purpose, the patient must *seem* an unwitting and involuntary victim of his malady. The unconscious purpose of the breakdown can be discovered only by a keenly-trained, impersonal observer who, sitting on the side-lines, as one might describe it, can see both the strategy of the patient's life and his personality disaster in their proper perspective. For the patient the breakdown is but a nightmare of suffering. And this suffering has a peculiar quality which we have already indicated in the foregoing chapter. Just as the courageous individual musters almost superhuman powers when faced with a critical test, so the individual with the nervous breakdown musters superhuman suffering to meet his critical needs.

It is for this reason that every patient with a nervous breakdown has " unheard of " symptoms, " intolerable " anguish, " unbelievable " pain, " torturing " doubt, " unprecedented " indecision, " besetting " fears, fantasies " beyond human belief ", " unspeakable " obsessions, " inhuman " suffering. When the psychiatrist tells the patient that there are others in the world who present the same complaints, he is put down by the patient as a fool or as an unsympathetic clod. " Why, doctor," says the patient, " it is inconceivable that anyone should go through this suffering. You have never seen a case as bad as mine." The patient with a nervous breakdown is usually extraordinarily resistant to sedatives, and frequently the physician who "cures" one symptom by heroic medical measures is rewarded for his pains by finding that the patient has produced another symptom more intolerable and more torturing than the first. Small wonder, then, that the general practitioner, unversed in the virtuosity of the nervous patient, gives up in despair when two new symptomatic dragons arise from the gore of each symptomatic dragon he has slain!

THE DECALOGUE OF THE NERVOUS BREAKDOWN

The symptoms of the nervous breakdown obey the decalogue of all neurotic conduct, and in a true nervous breakdown are characterised by the following fundamental attributes: 1. The patient must be *unaware* of the meaning of his symptoms. The symptoms must *seem* beyond his control, and they must indicate a basic lack of social co-operation. 2. The symptoms must indicate a basic egocentricity. The patient must be convinced of their uniqueness if they are to retain their value in the *gestalt* of his nervous breakdown. 3. The symptoms must occur either during a critical situation, just before, or just after it, and must be surcharged with an unconscious fear of an impending personality disaster. 4. The symptoms must effectually establish a subjective and emotional sense of security, whether this security derives from a feeling of power, a feeling of abject helplessness, or a feeling of moral superiority which is expressed in the unconscious indictment, "See what you have done to me!" 5. The symptoms must attain, or approximately attain, the goal of "face-saving". 6. The symptoms must effect their goal by establishing the patient's physical helplessness, and simultaneously evince his *conscious* willingness to face the problems which he is *unconsciously* avoiding. The symptom of the nervous breakdown is an unconscious "arrangement", a piece of unconscious legerdemain in which a painful, often intolerable "I cannot" is substituted for the even more intolerable admission of "I will not because I am afraid of losing 'face'." 7. The symptom of the nervous breakdown must establish a scapegoat. This scapegoat serves to divert the world's (and the patient's) attention from the actual situation. This scapegoat must appear to be entirely beyond the patient's conscious control. It may be a pain, an obsession, a doubt, an uncontrollable fear, or the like. The formula for the scapegoat is: "*If* I didn't have this pain (or obsession, or unfortunate fear) I would go on!" The scapegoat may sometimes be discovered in the rhetorical question, "How can you expect a man who *cannot sleep* to do his work?" The theme song of every nervous breakdown begins with the words "if" or "but". 8. The symptom must seemingly lie outside the patient's voluntary responsibility. If the patient were to admit his responsibility in "arranging" the symptom, it would completely lose its value as a defence, and would lay him open to indictment of bad manners or malingering. 9. The symptom must be futile, and completely devoid of any common-sense foundation. It is always exaggerated in intensity, and is based on the patient's "private logic" rather than on accepted common sense. 10. The symptom must either effect the patient's isolation from the open competition of his fellows, or it must effectually limit his sphere of activity to a constricted and futile "side-show" of life. The patient with the nervous breakdown is so busy fencing with the ghosts of his own creation, that he has neither the energy nor the time to face the objective problems of existence.

THE BODY SPEAKS: "ORGAN JARGON"

The particular constellation of symptoms which we find in any given nervous breakdown depends upon a variety of factors. In the first place, the symptoms are relative to the patient's physical constitution, and they especially depend upon minor functional anomalies of his tissues and organs. It is a well-known law of medical psychology that an inferior organ or organ-system frequently becomes the "loud-speaker" which broadcasts the protest of the individual as a whole. We can broadcast our panic with our hearts or intestines as well as with our words. This is indicated by the variety of physical manifestations of fear. Some individuals cannot catch their breath when they are afraid, and some cannot digest their food. Some men tremble or have goose-flesh, while others experience an urgent desire to urinate or to empty their bowels. Certain men are " paralysed " by fear, others exhibit frantic activity, some cannot swallow, and others vomit; and certain types of men and women experience great sexual excitation when they are afraid. We call these physical manifestations that accompany fear " organ jargon ".

There are more ways than one of saying " I am afraid! " In the nervous breakdown physical manifestations of fear are exceedingly common. In those individuals who have by nature a sympathetic nervous system which is easily disturbed in its equilibrium, the most fantastic physical symptoms may be present. Thus the psychiatrist hears of " terrible " tearing of the heart, " an unholy jumping " in the stomach. Patients complain of being " all choked up " or of feeling " hot and cold shivers " running up and down the spine. Headaches, usually centred in one part or one half of the head, always of the " splitting " or " nerve-racking " variety, are common. A general feeling of uncontrollable " jumpiness " occurs at some time or other in almost every nervous breakdown. In one case the patient indicates his helplessness by fatigue, apathy, lassitude, and insensibility, and in another there is an uncontrollable desire to " keep moving ", " racy feelings", "churnings ", " tearings ", " fidgets ", and the like. In each case the meaning is the same: " I cannot go on with these unbearable symptoms! "

Alfred Adler has pointed out that many sufferers " make " their symptoms unconsciously by swallowing air. The classic picture of aerophagia is that of the timid lover gulping air before he attempts to propose marriage to his beloved. This aerophagia distends the stomach, disorders the digestion, often pushes up the lining of the heart, causing palpitation and " fluttery " feelings, or it may push down the other viscera, giving rise to " sinking " sensations in the abdomen. Whatever the symptoms, or whatever their combination or sequence, the careful observer will find that they fit into the decalogue that governs all neurotic manifestations.

EMOTIONAL SYMPTOMS IN NERVOUS BREAKDOWN

The second category of symptoms is found in the emotional sphere. The emotional symptoms are as varied as the physical, and perhaps even more stubborn. Sedative pills may occasionally relieve a " splitting " headache, or still a " jumpy " heart, but there are as yet no pills for the " blues ". " Blues " and depressed feelings may alternate with agitated anxiety, anger may change to shame, and remorse and apathy to self-castigation, all in the same case of nervous breakdown. Often the boundaries between emotional and physical states are extremely difficult to determine. It must not be forgotten that the nervous breakdown is essentially a "face-saving" device that requires a well-organized offensive-defensive strategy. The patient mobilises all his psychic ammunition, often utilising such lightning shifts in attack and defence that the physician, the family, and the patient himself are utterly confused and disorientated. No matter what the manifestations may be, the emotional tone underlying all symptoms of a nervous breakdown is that of hopeless pessimism and stubborn non-co-operation. Every patient with a nervous breakdown is like a little Gandhi, dominating a small universe by the sheer force of his inertia and passive resistance.

If you would understand your own nervous breakdown, or that of another, stop your ears as did Ulysses passing the Island of the Sirens, and observe only the pantomime of the patient's conduct. If you are depressed, you give everyone in your environment the task of animating and encouraging you. If you are irritable or "jumpy", you present your entire environment with the problem of how to soothe and reassure yourself. If you are torn by remorse and insist on self-humiliation, renunciation, self-castigation, your self-sabotage has but one meaning: that someone else has to pick you up and put you together again.

Most individuals who suffer from a nervous breakdown have tried, at some time or another, to play the part of God—and have failed. It is part of the credo of every nervous breakdown to insist on an " either—or ", either an exalted, superhuman, god-like pre-eminence, or an infra-human, bestial, degraded, and despised inferiority. Raskolnikov, the inspired neurotic in Dostoievski's *Crime and Punishment*, puts it neatly when he asks the eternal question of the nervous breakdown, " Am I Napoleon . . . or am I a louse? "

In nearly every nervous breakdown, the patient at some time or another assumes an unconscious training which puts him in the class of the despised and rejected of the earth. Unconsciously he heaps abuse upon himself, declaims his utter worthlessness, and laments his complete incompetence. But when we examine this conduct objectively we discover that he does not mean it, and resents bitterly being taken at his word. The real meaning of his emotionally-arranged inferiority is to be found in his query: " What can you expect from a worm like me? "

HOW THE SYMPTOMS ARE CHOSEN

The unconscious choice of symptoms depends primarily, as we have said, upon the patient's own physical and emotional make-up, but it derives also from the nature of the critical situation, the patient's education, and the nature of the environment in which the breakdown occurs. All these factors must be taken into consideration in evaluating and treating the symptoms. Suppose a young woman who has always been pampered by her mother faces the necessity of getting married. She fears the responsibilities of her new position, the dangers of sexual relations, the difficulties of living away from her adoring parents, and finally the possibility that pregnancy and child-birth may damage her figure. Verbally she claims she is in love with her fiancé and is delighted with the prospects of marriage, and its attendant social and emotional liberation from the solicitude of her mother, but in the depths of her unconscious she fears that she is about to lose the paradise of her childhood.

Let us take the case of a young woman whose fiancé is a young and matter-of-fact surgeon who is very unsympathetic to minor, non-surgical ailments, and whose mother, on the other hand, is a confirmed valetudinarian who has always watched with an eagle eye for the appearance of the least symptom of a cold. She has kept her daughter in bed for weeks because of some indefinable malaise. We can almost predict the form of the nervous breakdown in this case: stubborn insomnia, which resists her fiancé's pills, "splitting" and uncontrollable headaches that enlist her mother's solicitude, combined with passive resistance in the form of doubt, indecision, and procrastination which will finally wear out her fiancé's patience. It would be useless to arrange anything else: the symptoms are exquisitely suited to the critical situation, her own physical constitution, and the nature and attitude of her environment. She accomplishes her unconscious purpose (the avoidance of marriage), neatly maintains her "face", adroitly shifts the responsibility for her failure away from herself, and finally, in receiving the complete exoneration of her family, she re-establishes her sense of security in the accustomed shadow of her mother's hearth.

A third category of symptoms falls in the intellectual and moral spheres. Fashions in nervous breakdowns change with the times, even as fashions in clothes, entertainments, or furniture. In the nineteenth century a young woman, who to-day would suffer a discreet nervous breakdown, probably would have had a major hysteria, with convulsions, paralyses, speechlessness, or even blindness. To-day such major hysterias are seen but rarely, and the probability is that the symptoms of a twentieth-century nervous breakdown will be more subtle and more effective. Among men and women of education and culture, the symptoms of the nervous breakdown are far more frequently found in the intellectual and emotional spheres, although the nervous breakdown is no respecter of class or culture, and its manifestations, either in form or in content, are seldom predictable.

THE RÔLE OF COMPLEXES

In the intellectual and moral spheres the nervous breakdown usually takes the form of what, in psychiatry, is called a complex. A complex is a form of unconscious strategy dominated by a definite emotional tone, in which a single stimulus gives rise to a complicated succession of acts, ideas, or feelings. The patient recognises the fact that his reactions are without basic foundation, but he cannot rid himself of the compulsion to occupy his mind with them. Some of the commonest forms of these complexes are worry, preoccupation with unwanted ideas, obsessions, a sense of personal persecution, compulsion, vague anxieties, and the like. It is impossible even to catalogue the symptoms that fall into this group, because any conceivable neurotic symptom may be the apex of the pyramid of the strategy of the nervous breakdown. The symptoms must, however, lie outside the patient's insight or awareness, and must accomplish its unconscious purpose.

Let us take a case of neurotic worry as an example. A young woman who has always devoted her life to the pursuit of pleasure, with no regard to the rights of others and no sense of her own social responsibility, forges a cheque to pay for a gambling debt. Her private, personal logic is so ingrained in her that she does not give a second thought to the clumsiness of her forgery, and believes that, if she says nothing about it, it will pass unnoticed and that this childish evasion of reality will serve to discharge her unpleasant obligation. The matter of the forgery is quickly discovered, and as a result her lover, whose name she has forged, refuses to see her any more, and withdraws his customary support from her. In the course of the legal investigation of the forgery her employer learns of the dishonesty, and she is threatened with the loss of her position. This is a difficult situation for anyone, even for a young woman who has been accustomed to riding rough-shod over the feelings and opinions of her fellow men. Her sense of " face " is threatened, and she is in an actual panic lest her entire unwholesome style of life collapse. Critical measures are required in this critical situation.

Immediately after the discovery of the forgery, the young woman suffers a profound sense of depression. In her panic at the thought of losing both her lover and her position, together with her fear of a possible criminal prosecution, with the consequent loss of " face " among her associates, before whom she had always played the false rôle of a *grande dame*, her mind becomes confused. She begins to forget names and dates, and makes silly mistakes in carrying out the orders of her employer. She breaks into tears at the slightest provocation. She complains of " terrific " pains at the back of her head and at the base of her spine. Her expression is sad, her usually jaunty gait has degenerated into a slouch, and she is no longer cheered at the thought of an invitation to the theatre. Clothes have lost their appeal, she neglects her hair and finger nails, smokes one cigarette after another, and gives the general appearance of dejection and despair.

One morning she awakens with a pain in her breast. She immediately makes the mental diagnosis of cancer. The word cancer obsesses her all day long, but she is afraid to consult a doctor. It seems suddenly as though cancer were the one subject of conversation on everyone's tongue. She cannot sleep for worry, and at every opportunity she retires, feels her breast, and imagines that the painful breast is growing harder and larger than the other. After a week of ceaseless torment she confides her fears to a friend who takes her to a doctor. The most elaborate examination reveals that she has not the slightest evidence of cancer. She sleeps for the first time in weeks.

HOW THE COMPLEX WORKS

On the following day she meets an old friend and companion of her gambling days. She does not recognise her at first. The friend, astonished at the obvious rebuff, chides our patient for being " superior ". The patient looks at her in blank amazement. She remembers the girl's face, but cannot recall her name. She gulps, excuses herself, breaks into tears, and runs away. A feeling of unreality seizes her. She pinches herself to see whether she is alive. Her mind is confused, thoughts crowd in furious sequence. The picture of a beggar stretching out a deformed hand to her dominates her mind. The thought, " I am going mad! " obsesses her. She strokes her forehead as if to wipe it away. The more she tries to divert her attention, the more the words "Crazy! Crazy! Going crazy!" flash through her mind. Hot and cold flushes pass like lightning down her spine. Her hands become numb, when she looks at herself in the mirror her eyes appear lifeless. She tries to test her sanity by remembering the telephone number of her former lover. She rushes to the telephone and dials the number. By some curious chance of fate she has called an undertaker. A new fear mounts in her mind. "I'm dying!" she shrieks, "I'm dying!" As the telephone receiver slips from her hands she falls to the floor in a faint.

Her employer summons his chauffeur and has her taken to a nursing home. Her mother is notified, who, knowing nothing of the circumstances of her daughter's difficulties, summons the girl's former lover to the nursing home. The employer sends flowers, the former lover comes to her bedside, relatives ply her doctor with gratuitous advice. In the panic of her complete prostration the matter of the forgery is temporarily forgotten. The good-natured doctor, seeing only the physical evidence of overwork and hard living, prescribes a long rest and then, if possible, a sea voyage. The former lover, moved by her pitiful plight, agrees to foot the bills for her care. She has gained her unconscious goal: the restitution of the false paradise of her pampered youth in which she may play the charming rôle of a sick, beautiful, and completely irresponsible Eve.

We must not suppose that this young woman

comprehends this sequence of events as we have described it. She suffers and has suffered agonies. The flowers, the rest in the nursing home, the sea voyage, the attention of her former lover, the solicitude of her employer are of no avail. She remains blue and depressed, and thoughts of death and insanity torture her still sleepless nights. She is caught in the toils of her own unconscious mechanisms. Weeks pass into months. The breakdown which rescued her from an impending loss of "face" is now her tyrant. The cry of despair which compelled her old worshippers to come to her side has become a chronic lamentation. At the first signs of impatience on the part of her family and friends her despair deepens. She has lost her way and her hope.

This characteristic picture of the course of a nervous breakdown not only demonstrates the workings of emotional and intellectual complexes, but also shows the relationship of the complexes to the patient's "organ jargon." Despite the unusually difficult circumstances surrounding this case, the young woman not only recovered completely from her breakdown after a psychological re-education, but is now launched upon a common-sense career as a wife and mother. She looks back upon the hectic experiences of her breakdown as one would look back to a bad dream. Her present happiness is based on a common-sense attitude toward life. As part of her compensation for her former vanity and thoughtlessness, she devotes much of her spare time to the care of poor children in a day nursery. Her entire pattern of life has undergone a radical change, and in her new pattern her time is so filled with useful occupations that a recurrence of a breakdown is practically excluded.

UNCONSCIOUS STRATEGIES IN NERVOUS BREAKDOWN

Certain types of conduct are so common in the nervous breakdown that they merit further description. These are characteristic strategies of evasion. They are hesitation, indecision, doubt, procrastination, passive resistance and self-sabotage. It is obvious that all these types of conduct serve to forestall any basic test of the personality. The individual with a nervous breakdown unconsciously attempts to postpone the day of final judgment, the ultimate test of his personal " face ". We have seen an executive who had the fate of four thousand employees in his hands, whose financial judgments had been highly esteemed by his associates, spend three hours in the choice of a tie, and then finally slump to a couch in utter despair at his inability to choose between a grey and a blue one.

Another business man who suffered from a breakdown suddenly became suspicious that his food was poisoned. He would discharge his cook and engage another after endless inquiries and examination of references. The same procedure followed. The result was that he spent so much time over his meals that he was unable to go to his office, where he feared the evil consequences of a bad investment would result in his dismissal from the board of directors. This technique we call "lying with the truth". The patient unconsciously "stacks the cards" against himself, and then when he has lost the game, he truthfully says, "You see, I am a miserable player." But the process of *stacking the cards* is carefully hidden in the depths of his unconscious.

SELF-SABOTAGE

It is not uncommon that some friend or member of the family of an individual suffering from a nervous breakdown gives him some sound common-sense advice. The patient, with a certain degree of insight, tries to demonstrate his good will, but follows the advice in such a fashion that his condition is worse than it was before. He implies: "You see, I tried to take your advice, but look what has happened to me as a result!" We call this mechanism self-sabotage. It is like somebody cutting off a hand to prove that they cannot write an unpleasant letter. Self-sabotage is an extremely common device, but its manifestations are so subtle that they elude all but the trained observer.

In the moral sphere, self-sabotage is sometimes accomplished by obsessions which put the patient in an unfavourable moral light. Thus, a Baptist minister who suffered from a breakdown because he failed to interest his congregation with his sermons, was obsessed with all manner of filthy words and obscene phrases. Try as he would, he could not divert his attention from them. No sooner did he succeed in getting the words out of his mind than lewd and obscene picture and images crowded into his consciousness. This is one of the best examples of self-sabotage, the meaning of which becomes clear in the minister's answer to the psychiatrist's query, " Why don't you get back to work in your church? " The patient promptly answered, " How can a man with such filthy words in his mind and such lewd pictures in his imagination preach the Gospel of Christ? " It was " face-saving " at a terrible price. The patient had to prove his unworthiness by degrading himself to the lowest depths. There is no escape from the irrefutable conclusions of such " private logic ". Self-sabotage is the crystallisation of the process of " lying with the truth ".

SUICIDE AND THE SUICIDAL IMPULSE

The final degree of self-sabotage is suicide. There is hardly a nervous breakdown in which the thought of suicide does not occur at some stage or other. Self-destruction is one effective method of avoiding a difficulty or a test of " face ", but it is a very costly and drastic one. Death is absolutely final. It permits of no post-mortems except those of the pathologist. In Vienna there is a club for those who are about to commit suicide. Anyone with a suicidal impulse is eligible. No attempt is made to deter the member from his purpose, but he is given the opportunity of talking over his troubles with a sympathetic person. More than eighty per cent of those who come with self-destruction in mind leave with a more courageous point of view, and decide to go on with the struggle of life. Many coming to the club find, in talking with other prospective suicides, that their own situation is not nearly as bad as it might be. For some, the suicide club offers the first opportunity for social contact, and the fellowship of other miserable spirits in itself makes life worth while to many members. Not infrequently, one candidate for suicide discovers that he can assuage the agonies of another, and in finding himself socially useful again loses the impulse to do away with himself. Suicide seems to be a very drastic method of demonstrating one's incompetence, especially when a few words of counsel and advice may serve to clarify the potential suicide's whole point of view, and open the way to an effective adjustment to reality.

In some cases, suicide represents a drastic revenge. The suicide attempts to justify his self-destruction with specious moral camouflage when he expresses the belief that those he leaves behind him will be better off when he is dead. He does not take into account the terrific mental torture that he bequeaths to those who remain behind to battle with the realities. Suicide after a disastrous love affair is a not uncommon method of punishing an unattained lover. It is a lasting revenge which may leave ugly scars. "See what you have driven me to do!" the suicide says unconsciously, leaving the person he has made responsible for his own romantic failure the unwelcome legacy of a sense of guilt and remorse.

IS SUICIDE JUSTIFIABLE?

Does it require courage to commit the final act of self-sabotage? Suicide would certainly require superhuman courage from a normal person, but to the person with a nervous breakdown, whose judgments have become confused and whose values have become unsound, suicide is not an act of courage. Water flows down hill. Human beings take the easier course. There may be some few occasions when suicide is justifiable, but most suicides are justified neither by the facts alleged nor by the motives given, and certainly not by their after effects. In my experience there are very few occasions where suicide can save a tottering sense of "face". It seems preferable, therefore, to re-examine the facts in the presence of a sympathetic and understanding person. It is more courageous, really, to work out an adequate technique of life than to protest one's hopelessness and despair, and thus to perform the irrevocable gesture.

Many suicidal attempts are unsuccessful. These unsuccessful attempts are frequently unsuccessful because the individual who makes them is not at all desirous of carrying his self-sabotage to its threatened conclusion. He wants only to warn his environment of his delicate condition, thereby attaining a tremendous sense of power. "We must treat him very carefully! You know he has suicidal tendencies, and once nearly succeeded in doing away with himself!" say the members of the family. The nervous individual counts on this added solicitude, and succeeds in tyrannising his family or friends with his threats. Even stout hearts become solicitous under these circumstances, because no socially responsible individual wants to have the feeling that he is responsible for the suicide of a dear one, simply because he neglected to take common precautions. We have seen a whole family paralysed in its activities because one individual chose the threat of suicide as a symptom of her nervous breakdown. Here again we must reiterate that the patient is only dimly aware of the effect of the symptom, and actually suffers an agonising fear of committing suicide in a rash moment.

Another favourite device of the patient with the nervous breakdown is to doubt whether he can ever get well. "Yes, your advice is very good, doctor. If I had only known you ten years ago, I'd be on the high road to health. But it's too late now. I'm sunk. There's no hope for me! " This stubborn pessimism of the patient with the nervous breakdown is part and parcel of his sickness. It crops up in some form or other in nearly every case. It becomes a creed and is observed with an orthodox piety which often breaks the patience of family and friends. And yet a great many nervous breakdowns could be cured by time, without medicine or psychological re-education, without hope, and with practically no co-operation from the patient. For in time the critical situation passes, or at any rate appears less critical than it seemed at first. The dire personality disaster that the patient expected does not happen. The panicky defences of the patient are never attacked. Time, circumstances, and friends rescue the sufferer from his mistakes. He may get well in spite of himself.

L'ENVOI: SYMPTOMS ARE NOT ARGUMENTS

Notwithstanding symptoms and feelings, obsessions and doubts, suspicions and fear, indecisions and procrastinations, self-castigations and self-sabotage to the contrary, the nervous breakdown is itself only a symptom of a curable condition. *Symptoms prove nothing and they are not arguments.* Their sole interest lies in the fact that they indicate a healthy reaction to an unhealthy technique of living. They will often vanish spontaneously with time;

they will disappear more quickly if you will co-operate in their cure; they will not recur if you substitute a normal, objective, common-sense strategy of living for the subjective, private logic of your former mistaken patterns.

CHAPTER THREE

OF CASES AND CURES—PART I

Adolescent Breakdown: *The case of James K., a boy who found his critical situation in the difficult new ad-justments of university life. Challenged by the threat of being "sent down" from his university, he at-tempts suicide as a means of evading an intolerable admission of failure; is rescued, but suffers a nervous breakdown.*—Social Breakdown: *The case of Ruth G., a young American woman, the victim not only of her mother's social aspirations, but also of a childhood of parental coddling and pampering. She found marriage to a Harvard professor an intolerable betrayal of her romantic ideals. This is the story of a self-appointed princess who eventually finds happiness in hard work.*

The case of James K., a boy who found his critical situation in the difficult new adjust-ments of university life. Challenged by the threat of being "sent down" from the univer-sity, he attempts suicide as a means of evad-ing an intolerable admission of failure; is rescued, but suffers a nervous breakdown.

ADOLESCENT BREAKDOWN

THE scope of this handbook of help and self-help is limited, as its title implies, to those cases of breakdown in which the perplexed individual can do something about his situation himself. We do not, therefore, in our discussion of cases, include those important miniature breakdowns that occur in the nursery and the kindergarten, on the playground and in the classroom. In these unfortunate cases, which modern psychiatry is attempting to prevent by the introduction of child guidance clinics in all schools, the individual, be he a "problem child", a juvenile delinquent, a timid, whining "cry-baby" or a "mother's pet", is thrown upon the mercy and understanding of his adult environment. There is little he can do for himself without the help of some intelligent and sympathetic adult. But with adolescence and early adult life, the affected individual has usually gained enough insight to be able to understand something of the dynamics of his own situation. He has the important lever of intelligence with which he can pry himself loose from mistaken patterns of conduct, and consciously develop a more effective strategy of living. Our cases, therefore, begin with an undergraduate, James K., who has attempted to commit suicide after having been compelled to leave the university because of scholastic failure.

James K. is eighteen years old, the son of a physician in a provincial town. He is the eldest of three children. His childhood was marked by no serious illness, although he was always small and underweight. At an early age he showed signs of a highly imaginative mind and considerable artistic promise. He peopled his world with the fairies and wizards of his phantasy, and seemed disinclined to play with the other children of his age. He was cruel to animals and attempted to dominate his younger and more robust sister, but was constantly afraid of being punished by his father. James would do anything to gain the praise and attention of his mother, a gentle and sympathetic soul who did not always agree with the stern, authoritarian dictates of her husband. School was James's paradise. He learned to read while other children were still making mud-pies. He was a model child at school because he was not only afraid of the possible displeasure of his teachers, but he also realized that good school reports were his chief claim to immunity from his father's punishments. The family was almost equally divided in its loyalties. James sided with his mother; his two younger sisters were loyal to the father. James wanted to be a poet or a musician, while both the girls wanted to emulate their father and become doctors. James was always shy, timid, withdrawn, subject to fits of bad temper which punctuated long periods of wistful day-dreaming. Any psychiatrist could have recognised the signs of discouragement in his conduct, but his father, being a heart specialist, remained unaware of the boy's difficulties.

At the age of twelve James discovered masturbation spontaneously, and found in this habit a compensation for his failures in sports, and a pleasurable retreat from his conflict with his father. It also acted as a satisfying counterbalance to his marked deficiencies in science and mathematics at school. He was never instructed at home about sexual matters, but displayed an abiding curiosity about them. The day he discovered an old text-book of gynaecology and obstetrics among his father's discarded medical books was a red-letter day in his life. He hid this book in the attic which he called his " castle ". Here he kept his first poems, his stamp collection, and the pictures of beautiful actresses whom he worshipped from afar. The older he grew the more he became ashamed of his physical inferiorities and his incompetence in competitive sports, and the greater his shame the more he resorted to masturbation as a solace. When he matriculated from school he was already deeply introspective, inclined to periods of melancholy, given to abruptness and bad manners, surliness, mock superiority, egoistic self-conceit, vanity, and adolescent cynicism. He hated girls, and worshipped the unapproachable actresses of the screen who peopled his day-dreams. He had already lost close contact with his mother because, as he grew older, she became increasingly interested in her own social activities. He hated his sisters because they had advanced beyond him both socially and scholastically. In four years at school he had made the friendship of only one other boy, a cripple, toward whom he felt decidedly superior. He sensed his own superiority, and lost no opportunity to display his contempt of his fellows.

When the question of a university came up, James's father, realising too late that the boy suffered from the tension of the home situation, and that he was socially maladjusted, suggested a distant college which had the reputation of turning out virile young men. James left for college with many secret misgivings and fears, all of which were justified in the first dreadful weeks of adjustment, hazing, loneliness, and nostalgia for his " attic castle ". At college he was unknown and unnoticed. The pranks of second-year men offended his ego and humiliated him beyond words, especially as he came in for more than his share of " ragging " for the very reason that he was considered a " queer fish ". His work was a nightmare to him. He could not adjust himself to the different academic standards, although he had come up with a good recommendation from his school. A university demanded independence and initiative instead of blind obedience in the classroom. The objective difficulties of analytic geometry and calculus, in particular, seemed entirely beyond his comprehension, while the prevailing cult of athletic prowess made him seem physically more inferior than he really was. In all this university town there was no note of sympathy, in all this world of lectures and sport, there was not one chord harmonious to his introspective aloofness.

With the coming of winter, grey skies and dreary days added to James's pessimism. Other, wealthier, young men went on week-end excursions, or were invited to the homes of friends. He had no friends, and no money to leave the town. In the midst of his loneliness and disillusion he experienced for the first time in his life a great access of religious feeling, but after a few visits to local churches his cynicism triumphed over his psychic need for a substitute for the absent father whose dominant rôle he had never consciously realised. He began to feel listless and depressed. He began to wonder whether his long-continued masturbation was beginning to show belated evil effects. Hitherto he had laughed about the religious tracts describing the physical and moral degeneration that is supposed to follow as a result of this " private sin ", but now that he began to feel in himself the very symptoms that are described in these terrorising pamphlets, he began to have doubts.

There was no one whom he could consult. His doctor was a gruff and unsympathetic man, the Dean of his college was a forbidding figure, his tutor was himself an introspecitve, intimidated little man, dominated by a buxom, loud-spoken wife. He dared not write to his father and he feared to offend his mother. At another university his younger sister was carving out a fine record for herself, and had been elected vice-president of her year. The ghost of failure began to haunt him. Finally, at the end of the term, James K. was called into the Dean's room, told that his work was unsatisfactory, and warned that if it did not improve very markedly he would be sent down. James stood before the august mentor of college destinies, twisting his gown in his fingers, mumbling promises of greater effort. He hardly heard the Dean's questions. He could scarcely wait to escape from this supreme-Father of the college. Once out of the terrifying presence, James burst into tears, tears of self-pity, of remorse, of panic and disillusion. He rushed to his rooms, threw himself on his sofa, and sobbed and sobbed.

On the following morning the world seemed unreal through the fine snow that was falling. The chapel bells had a curious sound. They seemed to be laughing at him, as if they were rhythmically accusing him: "Failure! Failure!" His first tutorial was in mathematics, and he was the first student called upon to recite. He rose to give the required equation, became confused, stood speechless, and finally sat down, his mind utterly blank except for the echoing rhythm of the chapel bells' indictment "Failure, failure!" Someone else sniggered. Suddenly it seemed as if all the faces about him were laughing at him. He blushed. The laughter became more noticeable. He felt his neck getting red, his cheeks becoming flushed, his forehead becoming suddenly damp and cold with perspiration. He got up and rushed out of the room without any clear purpose in his mind. Once out in the snow again, he ran bareheaded and coatless through the streets of the little university town towards the river. It was a cold day, but he could feel only his flushed cheeks and his perspiring, hot forehead. At the edge of the river he hesitated for a moment. He heard the echo of the chapel bells dinning in his ears again, and covering his face with his arm, plunged deliberately into the icy waters.

Two passing motorists effected his rescue, and James K. was taken to hospital. His parents were summoned. He refused to talk, and during the convalescence from his immersion spoke disconnectedly, punctuating his speech with unmotivated laughter, grimaces of hate, and gestures of defence. As soon as possible he was taken home, and his connection with the university came to an end. The diagnosis was "nervous breakdown from overwork".

It was after he had finished with the university that I saw James K. and explained to him for the first time the meaning of his isolation, his fear of his sister's competition, his resentment of his father's authoritarian education, and his terror lest he fail to meet his father's demands of high scholastic attainments. The facts about masturbation were made clear to him, and the boy was convinced that his habit could have no possible deleterious effect upon his brain. The importance of social co-operation as a foundation of a sane life was made evident to James. A sympathetic tutor was found who clarified the mathematical problems and showed that mathematics was no insuperable dragon. After I had won James's confidence, a three-cornered conference was held with his father. Dr. K. admitted his errors in handling his son's education, and promised to attain a more sympathetic and co-operative relationship in future. In this conscious re-valuation of old values, James suddenly found that his father was a human being, not an avenging fury. The successful sister came home for her vacation and spent much of her time in intimate and revealing talks with her brother, and proved that his ideas about her were unfounded. He learned how his defensive methods of saving his " face " had alienated his sister's love. He discovered how, in being pampered by his mother, and then deserted, he had falsely come to believe that all people were false and insincere.

The emotional tension of the whole family was perceptibly lessened by these conferences. James was assured that his family's sympathy and love were indestructible. After his psychological re-education he was sent to a farm where he learned to ride on horesback and chop wood. He had been given courage again. It did not seem difficult to make friends with the farm hands, the farmer's wife, and the farmer's sons. He followed my advice and tried, every day, to do some little kindness to someone, just to establish the feeling that he could be useful as well as clever. He began to take chances, where he had always defended himself before. His introspective tendencies imperceptibly vanished.

After a summer on the farm James K. returned to his home a different human being. His psychological re-education had opened new worlds to him. He had discovered that an " attic castle " is not nearly so secure as the friendship of one's fellows.

He had learned that his failures, both scholastic and social, were chiefly the results of his own niggardly investments in social collaboration. Cynicism seemed to have become a little cheap. Somehow Nietzsche seemed less important now than being out of doors. The ghost of masturbation had been laid in its proper grave. In the fall he transferred to another university. His first act was to begin a spontaneous conversation with another freshman, which ended by James showing the boy how to decorate his room. He entered a competition for the university newspaper. Mathematics seemed interesting and not at all difficult. At the end of the year he returned home with an excellent scholastic record, a job as director of dramatics in a boys' camp, which he had obtained through his own efforts, and a new courageous outlook on life. The technique of nervous breakdown was gone, and a new technique of courageous living had been substituted. To-day, three years after the breakdown, James is associate editor of an undergraduate paper. He is engaged to his sister's greatest friend, and is collaborating with his fiancée in writing a novel. He has found in golf the answer to his athletic problems, for in this game a serene spirit is an important adjunct. He compensates for his inability to get very long drives by the deadly accuracy of his putting. "You don't have to be a giant to be a good golfer" he once wrote to me. "All that is really necessary is to keep your eye on the ball, and keep on keeping on!"

We describe this case in the hope that other college men, other young men and women beginning their business careers, or just tackling the other problems of being grown up, will find the common-sense therapy applied in this almost tragic case a guide to their own psychological clarification and self-realisation.

SOCIAL BREAKDOWN

The case of Ruth G., a young American woman, the victim not only of her mother's social aspirations, but also of a childhood of parental coddling and pampering. She found marriage to a Harvard professor an intolerable betrayal of her romantic ideals. This is the story of a self-appointed princess who eventually finds happiness in hard work.

Ruth G. met her husband at the Lido, in Venice. She was visiting the gay capital of the Adriatic with her mother. It was her first trip to Europe, and she was practising all the technical wiles that a young woman of good family can acquire at the best finishing schools, on the assembled suitors, foreign and domestic, who found the warm sun and the balmy air stimulating to romantic avowals. Ruth was on the crest of a long wave of social success. She was pretty, not too intelligent, but accomplished in the art of small talk. Her bathing pyjamas were the sensation of a sensational beach, her evening dresses the best that Parisian *coutourieurs* could drape upon her lovely body. She was the toast of the Excelsior Palace. An Italian prince had offered her his villa near Florence, and a Spanish ambassador had staked his ancestral castle at Mallorca for her hand.

This long wave of social success began with Ruth's playing a Chopin waltz at her public school graduation at Bucephalus, Ohio, where Max G., her father, was the owner of the largest steel mill and the president of the local bank. Ruth wore a dress of real lace at graduation, in open defiance to her father, who, having once been a junk dealer in Pittsburgh, had insisted that his daughter should be educated democratically at a high school. Her mother, who had social aspirations, insisted on at least this one evidence of affluence and power. Mrs. G. prevailed on her husband to let democracy stop with the high school, and Ruth continued her education in Virginia. Her commencement was the second triumph of her life: she was chosen Flower Queen. In her five years at finishing school she had completely lost the bourgeois accents of Bucephalus, had acquired the poise of a Virginia belle, had learned to down cocktails without wincing, to ride well to hounds, to drive her own sports car, to dress in the cosmopolitan manner, and to face the world with a certain insouciant bravado. Her trip to Europe, a graduation present from her adoring father, was a culmination of a long series of minor social successes.

Among her suitors at the Lido was a handsome, but rather bookish and shy, young professor of mathematics at Harvard, who was spending a sabbatical year among the glories of Italy. Ruth favoured the Spanish ambassador, but her mother who came of a stock that had always worshipped learning rather than wealth, a stock that had an almost instinctive fear of foreigners, tipped the scales in favour of the young professor. Mr. G. came to Paris for the wedding, beamed on the young couple, presented his daughter with a diamond bracelet, the cost of which could have bought, for one year, the services of the entire Harvard mathematical faculty, and departed with his wife for Bucephalus, congratulating himself on the happy outcome of all his ambitions.

The young couple went to Cambridge, Massachusetts, after a brief honeymoon in the Pyrenees. Ruth, now Mrs. T., found the cloistered atmosphere of Boston decidedly chilling. She was much more accustomed to cocktails than to the calculus. It seemed as though there were nothing in Boston but faculty meetings, mathematics meetings, mathematics papers to correct every night, mathematical articles that had to be written for mathematical journals. Her husband, in addition to being a mathematician was also a cellist. It seemed to Ruth that he was more interested in his cello than in anything else in the world. Even mathematics were not so important as a certain Bach concerto which he practised and practised over and over again. Monday nights were devoted to faculty meetings; Tuesday nights to the Mathematical Society; almost every Wednesday night there was a meeting of her husband's advanced seminar in mathematics; Thursday nights he coached two graduate students; Friday night they visited the dull wives of other faculty members; Saturday night she went to the Symphony which was her only chance to wear her evening dresses and her diamond bracelets, and then came Sunday night. Sunday night had become the *bête noire* of her existence because on Sunday night the Bach Chamber Music Club met at her home, and her husband with five or six other men spent the whole night playing interminable Mozart, Brahms, and Bach quartets and quintets in which she took no interest whatever. It seemed to her that her husband's chief joy in his wedded life was the fact that marriage had given him a large sitting room, a tremendous black grand piano (the gift of her mother), and beautiful cabinets in which to keep his hundreds of musical scores.

After three months of this almost mathematical progression of fixed nights, Ruth telegraphed her mother, and the glory of Bucephalus descended upon the arid intellectual wastes of Cambridge in all the splendour of a dun-coloured Rolls-Royce, personal maids and chauffeurs. The Bach Club went into temporary retirement for two weeks, bowing before the superior power of resplendent opera parties, night club evenings, and other extravagant entertainments. Ruth felt her old self again. She found herself talking almost ecstatically about her husband's " amusing " Bach evenings, about the unsophisticated professors and their frumpy wives, and the pleasures of being a " mathematical widow ". Boston tongues wagged. Ruth's husband began to wilt under the unaccustomed pressure of dressing for dinner, dining and dancing until the early morning, and teaching classes as usual. At the end of the second week of festivities he announced to his wife that he must be excused from the Opera that night to attend an important faculty meeting. Ruth made a scene. She would be disgraced if he did not appear with her. Her husband remained obdurate. For the first time in their married life they raised their voices. Ruth said some very unpleasant words about " not going to be a dowdy professor's wife! " The professor went to the faculty meeting. Ruth went to the Opera alone. During the intermission she wept in the ladies' room. Something seemed to burst in her—as if all the pent-up feelings of a lifetime had been suddenly liberated. Her heart began to pound. She felt dizzy. She sent the maid out for aspirin tablets and took three. Half the second act was over when she appeared again in her box. She seemed haggard, anxious, wan. In the darkness no one noticed her. She began to weep again. In the next box people were casting sidelong glances at her. She struggled to pull herself together, almost ran out into the street, and took a cab to Cambridge.

When she arrived home she was weeping bitterly. She felt betrayed. She was determined to " have it out " with the professor, but as she walked into his bedroom, her fists clenched, her eyes red, streaks of mascara on her cheeks, she was met by the peaceful spectacle of her husband sound asleep. The light by his bed was still burning. He was holding his tortoise-shell glasses limply in his hand. A pile of papers scribbled with mathematical hieroglyphics was scattered over the bed and on the floor. On the professor's sleeping face was an almost idyllic expression, as if he had just dreamed through to the solution of a difficult problem. It was too much. Ruth fled to her room. She wanted to pack her suitcase and go straight to her mother and pour out her troubles to that ever sympathetic ear. But she was too proud. She reached for a suitcase, and threw in a few articles of clothing, but none of the things were pressed, and, after all, the maid could pack them much better in the morning. She took more aspirin, and cried herself to sleep.

When she awoke on the following morning her head and her eyes ached, a band seemed to encircle her skull. The pain was as if someone were twisting a steel coil about her forehead. She could almost feel the sickening sensation of having her head cut in half by a steel cable. It was Sunday morning. Someone opened a door and she heard the familiar

Sunday morning sound of the professor's cello squeaking through the Bach concerto. That same phrase! Why didn't he ever play it correctly, or give up playing it forever? The familiar notes came up with the smell of coffee and frying bacon. Ruth felt nauseated. Her headache continued. She tried to ring for her maid. As she lifted herself up on her elbow, a fit of dizziness and nausea seized her. A thought flashed through her mind. " Maybe I'm pregnant! My God! " She fell back on the pillow. Escape would be impossible then. She began weeping again, and failed to notice the maid, bringing in the morning coffee. The maid called the professor. " The missus am gone hy-ster-ical! " she told him in horror.

When Ruth saw her husband in the doorway of her room she was overcome with revulsion. The nausea became worse. " For God's sake, get out, get out! " she screamed. " Get out, both of you! " The professor and the maid retired in confusion. A doctor was called in; he prescribed rest and sedatives. Only Ruth's mother was allowed in her bedroom. For three days Ruth wept almost unceasingly. She refused to speak coherently. The house was kept in absolute quiet. Husband, parents, and servants tiptoed and spoke in whispers. The cello was mute.

Any mention of her husband's name seemed to aggravate Ruth's condition, and the doctor advised him to move temporarily to the Graduate Club. The household was managed by Ruth's mother. The greatest specialists were called in. Only after a delicate biological test had proved beyond doubt that Ruth was not pregnant did she stop weeping. After the gynægologist had reassured her she seemed to brighten up. The professor returned home. Ruth seemed to have lost her feeling of revulsion for him. Her mother remained for a week to console her, and finally left for Bucephalus, assured that her daughter was on the high road to recovery. " She was always a sensitive and nervous child, you know," she said by way of explanation. " Just a tempest in a teapot! The first year is the hardest in all marriages."

Her mother gone, Ruth's condition took a new turn. Her doctor had prescribed long walks in the open air as a tonic. Ruth tried to follow his advice. She dressed herself warmly, and went into the street. For the first few hundred yards all went well. She felt her old self again. The wind was whipping her face and bringing colour to her cheeks. She stopped at an important cross-roads to wait for the traffic lights to change. Cars were whirling past her. She saw an old lady uncertainly attempting to cross the street against the traffic. The old lady was completely bewildered. A taxicab dashed around the corner and almost ran into her. Ruth was standing paralysed. A man rushed out from the pavement and caught the old lady by the arm and escorted her to the curb. The lights changed. People began to rush across the street. Ruth was rooted to the spot. She felt dizzy, nauseated, anxious. She started to cross. The lights changed again suddenly, and the waiting cars seemed to leap at her. She retired to the kerb. She felt faint. "If only someone would rescue me!" she thought. No one came. Her dizziness increased. It seemed as if the cars were swooping up and down mountains on either side of her. The pavement seemed to roll beneath her like the deck of a ship labouring in a heavy sea. Everything whirled and swirled before her eyes. Cars, people, buses, traffic lights, more cars, red taxis, yellow taxis, blue taxis—all were spinning in a mad kaleidoscope. She felt she would faint. With one last effort she clutched the arm of a man who was passing by. She did not know whether she was going to vomit or to weep. "Please, please, get me a taxi and take me home!" she pleaded, "I'm terribly sick."

The stranger held her, helped her into a cab, and brought her home. As the cab reached her door she suddenly felt better. She insisted on paying her own fare. She thanked the man and rushed into the house. In her bedroom she pulled off her hat. The pictures were whirling around the wall. Her forehead was covered with beads of perspiration. She seemed cold and clammy all over. She went to bed, the doctor was called, and the professor summoned from his classes. She did not feel easy until they were both standing in her bedroom. The doctor tried to dismiss the incident as unimportant. "Two days more in bed, my dear, and you'll be as fit as a fiddle!" he said cheerfully. The mention of the word fiddle sent a shiver down her spine. She remembered the pale-faced violinist in the Bach Club. " For God's sake, Harold," she implored her husband, " stay with me. I'm afraid, I'm frightened to death. You mustn't leave me, not for a moment! " And," she added as an afterthought, " never bring that Doctor Jones into this room again. I hate him. I hate his smugness! Please, please don't leave me, Harold! "

The professor pleaded a sick wife, and for two weeks remained at Ruth's bedside every night, and as much of the day as he could spare from his classes. Ruth seemed to improve perceptibly. They planned for another trip to Venice in the spring, as soon as the term was over. Everything would be all right. Then one fine day Ruth decided to go out to do some shopping. She took a cab to the store, but despite inner qualms she managed to get through her shopping. Then she was going to test herself. She would be brave and lay the ghost. She would walk home. For a bit everything went well. The next corner was a busy traffic intersection. What if she were to get dizzy again? What if she should have a " spell " right in the middle of the street and be run over by a taxi? Her throat became dry. She gulped. The steel band re-appeared about her head. The street began to whirl. She *was* dizzy.

Ruth hailed a taxicab, ordered the driver to disregard all traffic rules, and get her home as quickly as possible. The moment she got into her bedroom, the dizziness and fear vanished. She summoned her husband from his classes, and when he appeared, she began to weep softly. " You must never leave me, dear! " she cried, " I simply cannot be alone. The minute I am alone I become frightened and dizzy. I am terrified if I go on the street. You must stay with me here until I get well." And in effect, that is what her husband was compelled to do for three weeks.

The Bach Chamber Music Club was compelled to return to its dingy old quarters, and to find a new cellist. The Mathematical Society and the Faculty Club did not see Mr. T. once during those weeks. The freshmen under her husband's care were shifted to other tutors whose wives were not in the throes of a nervous breakdown. Ruth's condition improved, but she stubbornly resisted her husband's attempts to make her go out on the street. She did try going out during the first week of her relapse, clinging timorously to his arm. In the last week she refused to go out under any conditions.

It was only when the full-blown tyranny of Ruth's breakdown began to tell on Mr. T.'s own morale and on the quality of his professional work, that he insisted on a psychiatric consultation. Ruth's breakdown was given the scientific name of agoraphobia, the fear of open places and people, and a psychological analysis and re-education were recommended. The first step in the treatment was her removal from Boston to New York. She took up her residence with a school friend, and the preliminary analytic consultations had to be held in her home, as she refused to risk an " attack " on the busy streets of New York.

During these first discussions, Ruth confessed that she had always been a spoiled and pampered little princess and that her notions of love and marriage were culled chiefly from novels and magazines. She soon began to realise that her idea of marriage was infantile. She had expected that marriage would represent an improvement on the almost ideal life that she had led. She had expected that Boston society would fall on its knees before her. After several talks she recognised how she had always depended upon her mother for appreciation, and how she had lacked all spontaneity and initiative during her whole life. It dawned on her that the unconscious motto of her life had been " I'm a princess. If I am not treated as a princess, I will not live at all. I must be treated as a princess, no matter at what cost."

Only after weeks of painstaking disclosure of her past pattern of life did Ruth recognise that her breakdown had been a " face-saving " device. She had been unable to adjust herself to the demands of an altered social position in which she was quite obviously not playing the princess rôle. The realities of Boston had been a distinct deflation of the romantic promises of Venice. She saw how she had refused to co-operate with her husband, and how she had failed to interest herself in the new opportunities of her married life.

She recognised how, unconsciously, she had been

afraid of pregnancy and childbirth, because taking care of an infant would have compelled her to relinquish the life of pleasure which she considered her due. She could not have tolerated sharing her husband's affection with her child because her hidden, unconscious goal was to absorb *all* the affection and appreciation of her entire environment. Suddenly she realised why she resented her husband so much, and how this feeling had been elaborated, via the organ jargon of nausea, into an argument for keeping him out of her boudoir. She saw how her breakdown, by compelling her mother to come to her side and take care of her, had served to restore her old childhood paradise. She understood how her symptoms had re-established her as the undisputed queen of her household, and how her nervous breakdown had magically removed the necessity of an adult adjustment to her marital and social responsibilities.

Only after repeated explanations did Ruth begin to understand the unconscious dynamics of her behaviour. She realised, herself, that her agoraphobia was an unconscious device to focus her husband's entire attention on her during the day and night. It served to remove him from all his other activities, and make him into her willing slave. She understood, finally, why this particular symptom was so effective.

At home Ruth had developed the technique of maintaining the centre of the stage. On the street she was not so certain that she could play her rôle of the misunderstood and ailing princess. Agoraphobia, as if by the waving of a magical wand, kept the Bach Club out of her home, and her husband at her bedside. By means of this complex, she re-established her position as the queen of her home, and this was the only position she could tolerate in terms of her old unconscious patterns. In a sense, too, she saw how her symptoms punished her mother. She had wanted, in Venice, to be an actual duchess, and had deferred under pressure to her mother's choice. Now her illness would make her mother sorry for being responsible for her unhappy marriage.

After some weeks Ruth gained enough courage to come to my consulting room in a taxicab, accompanied by a friend, and soon afterwards she was able to come by bus, alone. Somehow courage and optimism had been communicated to her. After a time Ruth began to realise that one could not carry out the rôle of a misunderstood princess, without paying a terrific price for it in sickness and limitation of motion. With this realisation she began to look around for more objective spheres of activity. Under the guidance of an intelligent musician, she began to learn something about the charm of Bach, Beethoven, and Brahms. Her interest in travel and languages was made the basis of further study. She joined the Foreign Policy Association, and began doing some research work in international problems. She took courses in international law and associated herself actively in the work of world peace. Almost every day new avenues of activity were opened to her, and the harder she worked, the more her old infantile reactions fell away. One day the Director of her office praised a piece of research work she had done. She came to my consulting room that day with a smile on her face. " You have no idea how nice it is to find that one is really useful to a big cause like world peace ! " she said. " Why aren't we taught this with our spelling and arithmetic ? "

In due course she was able to return to Boston and to her husband. As she stepped off the train her husband asked her what she had in her suitcase that made it so heavy. " You'll never guess," she laughed, "but it's full of gramophone records. Some new Brahms recordings from Europe that you haven't got in your collection yet." She found that instead of being the sworn enemy of the Bach Club, it was much more fun to be the librarian of its music. "We're going to give a benefit performance next month," she announced. " We need funds to send a delegate to the Peace Conference in Geneva, and you young men have to contribute your share by giving a charity concert! " She arranged all the details of the concert herself, and was able to realise a considerable sum for her cause. The Bach Club, naturally, was so encouraged by her change of heart, that it gave the best performance in its history.

Presently Ruth discovered that a number of the seemingly frumpy dons' wives could be interested in studying international law. She started a course of lectures in her home, inviting various authorities to give intimate talks to her group on the nights when her husband was busy with his extra-curricular duties. These were so successful that someone suggested to her that she should organise a small lecture bureau, and use her contacts for the purpose of getting lecturers for other small groups. Mindful of my advice that anything which would broaden her sympathies, her responsibilities, and her social usefulness would be an asset in the ledger of mental health, she incorporated herself as a lecture bureau. The greatest pleasure she had ever experienced in life came in furnishing her own " office ", and having real business conferences with prominent authorities. And thus, in less than a year after a devastating nervous breakdown, the " misunderstood princess " was transformed into a normal, happy, responsible woman, who found far greater satisfaction in being grown up than she had ever attained in trying vainly to recapture the lost paradise of her pampered childhood.

CHAPTER FOUR

OF CASES AND CURES—PART II

Sexual Breakdowns—Sexual Ignorance: *The case of Luella D. is the story of a young woman whose nervous breakdown was the immediate result of abject ignorance of sexual hygiene. Marriage was the critical situation, the ignorance of her husband a contributing factor. Enlightenment of both partners effects the cure.*—About Masturbation: *The case of Warren O. illustrates a common type of nervous breakdown associated with worry and remorse over the practice of masturbation. Here the breakdown was a defensive measure designed to forestall a critical test of virility.* —Masculine Protest: *The case of Gladys T., an American woman, is characteristic of many women. She based her sense of " face " on her " sex appeal "—and lost. She had to save her " face " by being ill until she discovered latent personality assets during her psychological re-education.*—Romantic Breakdown: *The case of Helen R. demonstrates the evil consequences of gossip, and a rigid and romantic code of moral conduct. This case is especially significant because it shows how a previously " normal " person may suddenly meet a critical situation and react with a nervous breakdown.*—Homosexual Breakdown: *The case of Roland D. typifies the homosexual neurosis. Here a boy, unprepared to assume the normal sexual responsibilities of adult life, meets a confirmed homosexual who seduces him. Afraid of being involved in a homosexual life, Roland has a nervous breakdown. Psychological clarification brings him the peace and enjoyment of a normal heterosexual marriage.*

SEXUAL BREAKDOWNS

NERVOUS breakdowns with a sexual basis are among the commonest forms of breakdown that occur. The reason for this is not difficult to find. Of all the problems that a human being must solve —the social, the occupational, or economic, and the sexual—the sexual problem is the one that requires the highest degree of courage, objectivity, training in social co-operation, and psychological maturity. A boy can earn his living at the age of fourteen selling newspapers, and a woman may find social solace at her parents' fireside, but the correct solution of the sexual problem, which includes mature love and the willingness to assume the responsibilities of marriage, a home, and children, requires and demands not only a certain degree of artistry, but also adequate preparation and training.

In addition to the existing difficulties, our education for the solution of the sexual problem is, with a very few exceptions, the least objective of all our educational efforts. Our children are taught the intricacies of algebra and they are compelled to master the military strategy of Cæsar's Gallic Wars, but practically nothing is taught them about the so-called " facts of life ". No one goes to a university to learn how to be a good husband or wife, or to take a course in the art of love. The more our educational institutions are silent about sexual matters, the louder do our unofficial educational institutions, the newspapers, the magazines, the cinema, popular novels and short stories, broadcast misinformation on sexual topics. Unfortunately, these unofficial sources of sexual education are, almost without exception, notoriously inept teachers. From the downright pornography of the " gutter Press ", the sickening sentimentality of infantile films, the psychopathological pruriency of the cheaper magazines, little honest light is offered to the individual who searches for knowledge and guidance in the sphere of sex. Honest, scientific books on sex often go begging for publishers, while the most outrageous trash finds a ready sale.

The third reason for the frequency of nervous breakdowns in the sexual sphere is a psychological one. The first overt signs of a nervous breakdown to appear are often sexual symptoms. You fail gradually in business and are almost unaware of the process. You isolate yourself from your fellow men, and no one criticises you very severely. But a sudden failure in sexual desire or potency is a dramatic event which is likely to send you hurrying to the doctor. " Face " depends in a large degree upon the ability to gain the love and appreciation of a member of the opposite sex. The almost universal belief in the power of love causes men and women to look upon it with romantic awe. They fully expect that successful sexual relations will magically cure their social or occupational irresponsibilities.

How often we hear someone say, "What he needs is a good wife!" or "All she needs is a good husband, and she'll be all right!" There is an almost universal belief that there is some inherent magic in sexual relations. Love is a task for mature individuals. Love between two mature individuals glorifies their social and occupational collaboration. But sexual union between two romantically inclined adolescents, whether they are fifteen or fifty-five years old, is likely to bring their own personality inadequacies to a glaring focus. The process of "falling in love", in the accepted sense of the word, is probably a neurosis in itself, and the unions that result from such a neurotic process can hardly be anything but neuroses. Because of these factors, "falling in love" is often the highroad to a nervous breakdown.

Ignorance of the art of love is another broad avenue leading to personality disaster. Competition between the sexes, based on the supposed inferiority of women and the desire of men to prove their alleged superiority, is yet another source of nervous breakdown, because happiness in sexual union can result only from sexual co-operation, never from a struggle for sexual prestige. Such great emphasis is placed on sex in contemporary society that many men and women seek falsely to establish their sense of " face " solely upon their sexual virtuosity. This leads to various forms of what I have called " sexual athletics ". A man who is a failure in every department of his life will often support his " face " with the belief that if he can seduce a woman he is " still a man ". A woman, likewise, who is a failure as a human being, often spends her life proving that she can make " men fall for her ", with inevitably tragic results. " Face " cannot be built on sexual virtuosity alone. Now let us examine some typical cases and show how these theoretical considerations work out in actual practice.

SEXUAL IGNORANCE

The case of Luella D. is the story of a young woman whose nervous breakdown was the immediate result of abject ignorance of sexual hygiene. Marriage was the critical situation, the ignorance of her husband a contributing factor. Enlightenment of both partners effects the cure.

The case of Luella D. is characteristic of a type of nervous breakdown which, happily, is not so frequent as it used to be. Luella D., the youngest of three children, was brought up in a strictly religious home. At the age of twenty she was only dimly aware of the physiological processes of coitus, pregnancy, and childbirth. Her ideas of love and marriage were gained chiefly from films and cheap novels, which she hid under her pillow lest her mother discover her reading " forbidden fiction ". She never matriculated in the crude but often efficient " gutter school " of sexual information, because she was a " good little girl " and carefully kept all thoughts of " nasty " subjects from her mind. At the age of twenty-one she was not quite certain whether a girl could get a baby by merely being kissed by a man, and she had never had the temerity to ask for fuller details. Born and bred in the city, she never witnessed the copulation of animals, and was thus unable to draw any analogies. Luella went to church regularly, lived a very good if circumscribed life, comported herself very modestly at the few dances she attended, and at the age of twenty-five married a young man two years her senior. He lived three doors away from her and had known her all her life.

Everyone was very happy that Luella was going to marry such a nice young man, and only a few suspected that he had been the first suitor she had ever had. Sly jokes were cracked, jokes whose import Luella did not undersetand. She felt vaguely that marriage was a beautiful state, which would cure the restlessness she had experienced in the last few years. On the eve of her wedding she consulted her mother for advice about sexual relations, but that dear good lady was quite inarticulate, and not a little hurt. " That is for your husband to tell you," she said,

" and I am certain Bill will be a very good and considerate husband." And so Luella entered matrimony like a lamb being led to the sacrificial altar.

Bill *was* a good boy, if not inordinately clever. He had had some sexual experiences, chiefly with prostitutes, and usually while drunk. He had always suffered some remorse after these sexual escapades. He knew practically nothing about contraception. His own education in sex had been such that he looked on sexual relations as somewhat bestial and shameful, but, being a lusty and virile young man, his sexual appetite was stronger than his inhibitions, and he had often deviated from his high ideals and consorted with women of a low type. Some kind friend had told him that he should brook no resistance on his wedding night, that he would never enjoy sexual relations as much as he would on that occasion. He took his friend's advice seriously.

For Luella, away from home for the first time in her life, that first night of marital " bliss " was one of abject terror, of horrible disillusion, of psychic panic and excruciating pain. The nice boy who had taken her to dances seemed suddenly transformed into a disgusting satyr. Her two weeks' honeymoon was a nightmare. She lost ten pounds in weight, became irritable, restless, preoccupied, easily fatigued, and acutely unhappy. Bill, on the other hand, seemed to thrive on the experience. His bubbling good spirits served to annoy her the more because she was so abjectly miserable. Luella felt deserted by all the world. Marriage was a cheat. Her mother had deceived her by her silence. In the light of her experience the jokes of her friends took on a new meaning. She felt that she had been sold into virtual slavery. She hated Bill, she hated her mother, she hated her unkind friends, and most of all she hated the sexual embrace. She experienced none of the " wonderful feelings " that a married friend had told her about—there was nothing to marriage but pain and disgust.

Her parents and friends, who noticed how she had lost weight and how bitter and silent she had become, chided her and told her to " snap out of it ". Bill's continuous good humour was evidence to them that there was nothing basically wrong. But Luella became more and more silent. She refused to eat. Her head began to ache, she began to feel sick every morning. Her mother took her to the family doctor. He examined her, smiled, patted her on the back, and condescendingly told her, " Well, young lady, I hope it's going to be a nice big, bouncing boy! " It was as if the sword of Damocles had suddenly fallen upon her. She started to weep and refused to eat. Nothing would cheer her. She sat about idly while her husband tried to furnish their flat. She would not get out of bed, or dress, or go out of the house. No one could console her, and when her husband or her mother came near her she screamed at them, and often tried to attack them.

Despite her loss of weight, Luella became a veritable tigress. On one occasion she chased her mother from her flat, brandishing a bread-knife in her hand, looking for all the world like an impersonation of one of the Furies. In her mad pursuit she fell down a flight of stairs, cut herself severely with the knife, and injured herself to the extent that she had a miscarriage in the hospital the following day. The miscarriage seemed to calm her to some extent, but Luella continued her surly silence and her hunger strike. In this state, she was brought to me by her doctor.

During the first consultations Luella did little more than weep, but when she found that she was to be subjected to nothing more serious than a few sympathetic questions she unburdened her whole story. The young husband was called in and given advice as to how to treat a young and hysterical wife. The mother was forbidden entrance to her daughter's flat. The " facts of life " were gently taught to the patient. She was encouraged to put the best possible interpretation on her husband's clumsiness. Her recovery was immediately hastened by Bill's willingness to learn and to put his new knowledge into execution. In a few weeks Luella had regained her lost weight, and found that she could really enjoy love. It was not difficult for her to reconcile herself to being a wife, but to this day she still scowls when her mother comes to visit them. Nervous breakdowns can be cured, but psychiatrists cannot make angels!

ABOUT MASTURBATION

The case of Warren O. illustrates a common type of nervous breakdown associated with worry and remorse over the practice of masturbation. Here the breakdown was a defensive measure designed to forestall a critical test of virility.

While we are considering the effects of sexual ignorance we must include a discussion of the bogey of masturbation. Probably more misconceptions exist on this subject than on any other in the whole sphere of sexual matters. Masturbation is a normal experience in the life of every individual, but in the lives of neurotics it often plays a very critical rôle. Let it be said at the outset that 99.99/100 percent of humanity has at some time or another, consciously or unconsciously, indulged in auto-erotic practices. The likelihood, therefore, that it has the damaging effects ascribed to it by well-meaning but deluded alarmists is infinitesimal. Neurotics are very prone to make the practice of masturbation a central problem of their lives. Their logic runs this way: " If I can stop masturbation, I am a man. If I cannot stop it, how can I do anything else? "

The conscious control of the tendency to practice auto-erotic acts is neither a real test of " face " nor of so-called "will-power". If we could get at the true records we should almost certainly find that the vast majority of the world's really great men and women has indulged in this practice at some time or another. *Masturbation is the sex life of an isolated individual.* Isolated individuals, as we have shown, are especially prone to have nervous breakdowns because their sense of " face " has no objective basis. This does not mean that masturbation causes nervous breakdowns, "softening of the brain", lack of will power, indecision, pimples, loss of manhood, falling hair, or any of the thousand other human ailments which it is credited with bringing in its wake. Masturbation is only a *symptom* of a false strategy of life. It cannot, in and of itself, have any deleterious effect. *Much more damage is done by thinking about the evil effects of masturbation than by masturbation itself.* Parents, teachers, ministers and physicians who fulminate against this habit and inculcate a kind of sexual jingoism into young men and women should read the following case, and learn the possible results of their teachings.

Warren O. came to consult me because he was in a state of panic about the effects of his long-continued masturbation. He was 28, attractive, well set up, well educated in all but sexual matters, sensitive, generous, but very timid. He had just lost his job, and he was engaged to be married. Everything in the world was black. He was caught between the pressure of his fiancée and her family, and the moral suasion of his own family, but he felt he could not go through with the ceremony. Friends had promised him another job, and even the employer who had dismissed him had offered him his post back again if he would concentrate on his work. He was literally incapable of the slightest form of concerted effort. All night long he tossed in his bed, haunted by fears, a victim of his own self-castigation. He had shut himself up in his room and refused to see anyone or to answer any telephone calls. The word " masturbation " seemed to echo from all four walls. He felt people had only to look at him to see that he had been a chronic masturbator. And now he was afraid that if he married he would be impotent. At the thought of being impotent, his mind reeled and refused to function. He was caught as if in a fog of fear and unreality.

Sexual virility is, as we have remarked, one of the chief supports of the sense of " face ". As long as a man can maintain his sexual virility, he may console himself that he is " still a man ". The presentiment of the loss of this virility is a frequent cause for a nervous breakdown. So it was in the case of Warren O. He had not only read the tracts that were so common years ago, which luridly described the physical and mental disintegration attendant on masturbation, but both a schoolmaster and a curate had filled his mind with the dire effects of the habit. Warren felt compelled to lock himself in his room. He refused to see anyone. Every moment of his day was filled with a torrent of thoughts, in which remorse, self-castigation, self-abasement followed each other in rapid succession. This isolation of himself seemed the only course to take to protect himself from the critical situations of marriage, the intolerable admission of sexual impotence and the disclosure of his " bad habit " to the whole world. And he rationalised this escape from reality by telling himself that he could not victimise an innocent girl and make her bear the onus of his " wasted life ".

Here again the cure consisted chiefly of re-education. Warren O. learned that masturbation was practically universal, that it could not result in impotence, and that the well-intentioned tracts and admonitions to which he had listened in his youth largely, if not entirely, exaggerated the aftermath of masturbation. Courage and hope were infused into his flagging spirit. The meaning of his symptoms as a defence of his sense of " face " against the threatening critical situation was explained to him. Case histories of other similar cases were cited. With this new knowledge, and the assurance that he had not done himself any irremediable damage, Warren O. felt that a new life had dawned. In his own words, " I feel that a great load has been lifted off my chest. I feel like a new and cleaner human being. I see that sex isn't bestial, and that masturbation is just a bogey! " And so in due course he married his fiancée, was perfectly virile and potent, and within a year and a half of his marriage, found himself a proud father.

MASCULINE PROTEST

The case of Gladys T., an American woman, is characteristic of many women. She based her sense of " face " on her " sex appeal "—and lost. She had to save her " face " by being ill until she discovered latent personality assets during her psychological re-education.

We live in a man-made civilisation. Laws, institutions and opportunities for development are still made predominantly by men and for men. We call ourselves emancipated, but we still close the door of our highest offices to women, and we almost universally allot the worst drudgeries to their hands. In a patriarchal civilisation such as ours, it is inevitable that women should feel a sense of inferiority just because they are women. The fact that there is no basis for this belief in the inferiority of women, either biologically or economically, either psychologically or historically, does not alter the weight of prejudice and superstition which makes itself felt in the life of the individual woman. Most women, at some time or another, find themselves frustrated in their ambitions or their conduct by the prohibitions of our culture. It is an inescapable fact that the woman pays.

It is natural that women, sensing the fallacy of these man-made laws, should consciously and unconsciously rebel and protest against them. Some women protest openly by cultivating mannish habits of dress and conduct, and try to prove that they are "as good as men". Finding that men occupy the more advantageous positions in life, these women attempt to act "as if" they, too, were men, in order to enjoy so-called masculine prerogatives. Other women protest more subtly. Openly they avow the superiority of the male, but unconsciously they spend their lives tricking men into a position of inferiority. They use their alleged weakness to make slaves of the men who love them. To this end they acquire what I have called "an aggressive sex-appeal". "Sex appeal" is as strong a weapon as any other when properly used, and in our modern civilisation with its over-valuation of the masculine ideal, a great many women spend their lives making capital out of masculine vanity and concupiscence. Such women build their sense of "face" almost entirely upon their ability to make men "fall for them". They do not know love, in the mature sense. For them sex is the arena in which they demonstrate the virtuosity of sexual athletics.

Needless to say a true sense of "face" can be obtained only in sexual co-operation, not in sexual competition, and any woman who builds her sense of "face" only on her ability to make men her sexual slaves is in a very precarious situation. Sooner or later she will have to meet the critical test of being compelled to admit to herself that her one and only weapon for gaining significance has failed her.

Such was the case of Gladys T. Gladys was brought up as a very spoiled and beautiful child. She was so beautiful that her mother, who was herself very vain, lost no opportunity to show Gladys off to admiring male relatives and friends. Dress, looks, and clothes were always the most important thing in Gladys's life. She got through her career at school chiefly on the strength of her charm and prettiness. Girls either adored her, or hated her for being a " baby vamp ". She managed to survive her time at the university by making eyes at young lecturers. She was the most popular girl in her year and was invited to more house parties than any other girl in her class. Studies never interested her except when the instructor was handsome, but she was an expert in the art of make-up and a virtuosa in coquetry.

Everyone predicted that she would be married within a year of her first season after graduation. Gladys had been engaged three times during her university career, but each time she was about to announce her engagement a new man appeared on the horizon. He presented a challenge to her sex appeal and the chase was on again, while the current fiancé was quickly dismissed. Despite her reputation for fickleness, men continued to flock to her standard. " I hate my name," she once told an older woman, " I should have been called Diana. I am a born huntress, and men are my game. If a beautiful or an intelligent man comes along, I forget everything, and concentrate on snaring him. The bigger they are, the harder they fall. I won't stop until I win the Prince of Wales!"

If this older woman had only been a psychiatrist! She could have told Gladys that both her ambition and her vanity, not to say her methods of hunting, would lead to no good end. And once, indeed, Gladys did have an alarming premonitory experience. She met her male equivalent, a gay Casanova who bested her in the game of love, and left her before she had had a chance to give him his *congé*. For a week Gladys exhibited all the signs of a miniature nervous breakdown: sleepless nights, nervous indigestion, palpitation of the heart, spells of sobbing, depression, and a queer sense of futility and unreality. Mentally she made a reservation that she would study men more keenly, be more daring in her conquests, and more deadly in her heartlessness. She had learned nothing from her experience.

Gladys left home. She lived with men on three continents. She married twice, but found marriage equally irksome both times. Marriage had always been a concession to her final goal. She had found men whom she could not capture unless she married them. No sooner had she married them and made them dance attendance on her than she lost all interest in them, became sexually frigid, and promptly got a divorce. And now she was a divorcée, still rather pretty in a florid manner, still very apt at the game of love, still attractive to men. Men came and men went, but Diana never relinquished the chase.

Then she was hurt in a motor-car accident, broke her ankle, and was forced to remain in a secluded and inaccessible nursing home, far from any of her friends, for a period of three weeks. The doctors were old and unattractive. There were hours in which she had nothing to do but to think of herself. She began to examine her face. There were already tell-tale crows'-feet in the corners of her eyes, her chin was beginning to sag despite the excellent and frequent massages in which she had invested so many hours and so much money. Her dyed hair seemed suddenly ugly and dull. Her ankle hurt her. And the sights, smells, and stories of the hospital suddenly jolted her into the realization that she was growing old. In a few years she would experience the menopause, and she held the fallacious belief that with her " change of life " she would cease to desire men and no longer be attractive to them. Then the chase would be over, and nothing left for the huntress but the Old Ladies' Home—or suicide.

The ankle healed. Gladys went back to her home —but something had changed in her. She was never again the same care-free irresponsible woman. She grew querulous and irritable. She found herself nagging at her maid who had been her unflagging and devoted servant for eight years. She became economical to the point of meanness in her household expenses. Whenever she saw an old woman on the street she began to sob, and if she saw two young lovers sitting on a park bench she became furious both at them and at herself. Her friends noticed the change. "What's the trouble, Gladys?" one of them asked her at a party. "Are you growing old?" This was a shaft that touched her in the most vulnerable spot. She lost her temper, burst into tears, and left the party. And then began a last mad chase after men. They had to be young men—the younger and handsomer, the better. But the old magic was gone.

She started a round of visits to doctors—had her face lifted, submitted to innumerable gynæcological examinations, and discovered aches and pains in every part of her body. Sleepless nights followed, and once in desperation she attempted suicide by taking an overdose of sleeping medicine. When she recovered from this, a friend brought her to my consulting room, suffering from a typical nervous breakdown. She had lost her courage to live. She had lost her belief in her own sexual attractiveness, and had retained enough insight into her own condition to know that her recent preference for young boys just down from the university, young officers, young men on the Stock Exchange, and the like, implied the tacit admission that she had lost her charm and that men of mature taste were no longer interested in her.

Here we have the classical picture of a nervous breakdown as a result of a fallacious strategy of life. The background: a spoiled, beautiful, " only " child accustomed to attention, restricting her sense of values to her good looks. The goal: to be adored by the mighty of the earth, and to feel that she could humble the highest. The method: the asocial technique of capturing, enslaving, and then humiliating by virtue of her sexual charm. The critical situation: old age, sans charm, sans husband or children, sans assured social position, sans beauty, and sans satisfying prey. The technique of the nervous breakdown: " I am a very sick woman. *If* it hadn't been for that accident I would still be gloriously young. Men take advantage of a woman. Life isn't worth living anyway! "

Now Gladys had some personality assets along with her many deficits, and—as in every case of this kind—the psychiatrist attempts to build up the affected individual's sense of " face " on the foundation of the existing assets, If you happen to be suffering from a nervous breakdown now, sit down and before you forget it, with paper and pencil, obey that old injunction: count your blessings. Draw a line down the middle of the page, and put your personality liabilities on one side, as honestly as you can, and your personality assets on the other. You will be inclined to over-rate the liabilities, and underrate the assets—that being one of the symptoms of a nervous breakdown. Therefore, you must discount your liabilities by at least forty per cent, and increase your assets by the same amount. And then begin making the existing assets into bigger assets. And here is a psychiatric aphorism for you: *Take care of the personality assets and the deficits will vanish by themselves.*

This scheme was followed with Gladys after some of the more flagrant misconceptions of her strategy of living had been cleared away. And one of the assets that stood out most clearly was Gladys's devotion to her two prize Pomeranians. Gladys's love for these dogs was the one shred of social feeling that she had left. I impressed the fact upon her that no one would ever care for these two dogs as well as she did, and that therefore she had to relinquish all thought of suicide, at least for the time being, in order to take care of them. Why not return to the country, have a little cottage, take up the breeding of Pomeranians as a vocation and avocation? From this make contacts with other dog-lovers. Join the local Kennel Club. Exhibit her prize dogs. Attain significance through this activity rather than through the mere sexual conquest of men. Then extend her interest by doing social service work at a hospital for crippled children, thus utilising her own hospital experience as a basis of identification and interest. And by these means we succeeded in building up her social feeling.

It is true that Gladys accepted these ideas chiefly for a neurotic reason. As she expressed it, " The more I see of men, the better I like Pomeranians!" But one must not take such rationalisations too seriously. The important thing is to begin *doing* the normal thing. Normal *feelings* come afterwards. And that brings us to another mental hygiene aphorism: *Act as if you were normal, and you will be normal.* "I will do right when I feel better" is a neurotic argument, and logically invalid. No matter how much it hurts in the beginning, you must take the risk of trying to give yourself a chance to get well.

Gladys took my advice and began a new life. She subsequently passed through her menopause without any untoward incidents, because she was too busy with a new litter of Pomeranians to pay much attention to her change of life. And when I asked her for permission to publish her story she added these words to her assent: "And Doctor, I hope you will write this in your book for the benefit of all the young women with a Diana-complex like mine: hunting man-scalps is good sport but awfully hard on the nerves. And it doesn't pay in the end. A good husband in the house is worth two brokers on the wing. And that's straight from the heart of a woman who was a good huntress in her day!"

ROMANTIC BREAKDOWN

The case of Helen R. demonstrates the evil consequences of gossip, and a rigid and romantic code of moral conduct. This case is especially significant because it shows how a previously " normal " person may suddenly meet a critical situation and react with a nervous breakdown.

The case of Helen R. will interest you from a variety of angles: first, because it demonstrates the incredible damage that can be done by the gossip of a neurotic person (because gossip gives her a sense of power); second, because it shows that any life based on a rigid moral code is likely to end in a breakdown if this code (which has been accepted uncritically since childhood) is exploded by the facts of adult life.

Helen R. was a typical " nice " girl, brought up wth bourgeois morality, in a bourgeois family. She was compelled, by circumstances, to earn her own living and in the course of her business career she developed not only great business ability, but also a code of sexual morality even more rigid than that which her parents had taught her. Her chief goal in life had been to marry a man of professional standing, have several children, and settle down to a happy middle-class existence. Her dream was realized when she met a young doctor who seemed to answer her every desire. They were married, and worked together for a number of years in perfect harmony and amity. Helen was convinced that her husband loved her only, and she for her part was completely and whole-heartedly devoted to him.

After they had been married for three years, her husband was honoured by being invited to read a paper at a foreign medical congress. While Helen was heart-broken that her business did not enable her to accompany him on his trip abroad, she made no demur at his going alone, although some of her friends asked her jokingly how she could trust her husband in Paris. She kept a stiff upper lip, laughed at their innuendos and continued her work, certain that her husband would remain faithful.

One day, when her husband had been gone for more than a month, a well-dressed, elderly woman walked into her shop, and inquired for Helen, saying that she must talk to her personally. When Helen came from her office, the lady introduced herself, telling Helen that she had just come from Germany. She inquired whether Helen was the wife of Dr. R., who was then in Germany. Helen was overjoyed, thinking that the lady would convey some greetings from her husband. " Why, you are charming, you are beautiful! " exclaimed the visitor, " I can't get over you. Stand up, let me get a good look at you! To think that such a delightful person . . ." Helen was somewhat puzzled by this unusual outburst. " My dear, I am sorry for you," her visitor continued, condescendingly, " I just *had* to come here, and look you up. I came here directly from the station. I simply *must* tell you that your husband, Dr. R., is carrying on the most outrageous love affair with a woman at a hotel in Carlsbad. And my dear, I could understand it if you were unattractive, but she simply cannot compare with you! I think you should know all the details," she added, drawing herself up with a show of moral indignation, fully prepared to unburden her insinuations to Helen's outraged ears.

Helen's heart was doing a tap dance on her diaphragm. She had been morally hurt. But she gathered her courage together, rose from the sofa, and said, " My dear Mrs. Brent, I do not care if my husband is having an affair with all the women in Carlsbad. That is his business, and I am not at all interested. But if you think that I am grateful to you for coming to me with your gossip, I am not. Good day! " Helen R., turned on her heel, and unceremoniously left her dumbfounded visitor sitting alone.

But the damage had been done. Helen looked up her husband's itinerary. He was to have been in Carlsbad for less than twenty-four hours. Was he travelling with a paramour? Was he losing all sense of the fitness of things? Had some smart Continental woman ensnared him with her wit and vivacity? Would he still return to her? What should she do? Her informant, judging by her manner, speech, and dress, was obviously a woman of some culture and sophistication. Was she reliable as a witness? These and a thousand other questions obsessed her for the rest of the day. She suddenly lost her appetite. Her love for her husband told her to disbelieve. Her knowledge of human nature compelled her to doubt. Her mind conjured up pictures of her husband in Paris, Biarritz, Nice, Bellagio, Stresa, Vienna, Carlsbad, Berlin—in each with a different lover. In her moral cosmos marriage was untenable when one partner was unfaithful. Divorce was the only way out, the only honourable way of saving one's face. But she was deeply in love with her husband. She wanted him back, she was lonely and disconsolate because he was gone. She was faced with an insoluble dilemma.

That evening she went to the theatre with friends. The play was a comedy, but in the middle of it she was compelled to leave them. She had broken into tears, which her friends at first thought were tears of laughter. She ran home to her flat. Her husband's photograph on the mantelpiece suddenly aroused her sense of hate. She wanted to throw it out of the window. She wanted to destroy every evidence of him. She took out his letters, and read them through, her rage growing with each word of endearment in his familiar bold hand, and burned them in the fireplace. As she looked into the flames she could see only images of her husband making love to a dreadful woman.

For a few days she went to her business as if in a dream. The whole world seemed unreal. There was no one with whom she could talk. Her family would certainly not understand. Should she wire her husband and demand that he return immediately?

Should she take the next train and go off in search of him? Should she take a lover herself, and show him that two could play at the same game? Should she file papers for a divorce action? How should she greet him on his return?

A terrible sense of shame, a sense of having been cheated, of having been betrayed, ran like a muffled melody throughout all these conversations with herself. One moment she had the impulse to go to the home of Mrs. Brent and kill her for having destroyed her happiness. Her pride and her good sense prevented her. At the next moment she cursed her husband for his infidelity.

Dreadful pains began to assail her. Her head felt as if someone were screwing a constricting steel band tighter and tighter. It reminded her of an old instrument of torture she had read about. She could not sleep. She had no appetite. Deep rings formed under her eyes; she lost her cheerful expression and assumed the aspect of a hunted animal. Her mind wandered constantly to the same theme: "I have been betrayed. Life is not worth while." Her physical condition became so bad that her business partner insisted she visit a doctor.

The doctor, a colleague of her husband, made a painstaking examination, and could find no organic basis for her pains. Elaborate neurological tests were made, because she seemed to show vague symptoms of a brain tumour. Helen had learned enough about medical symptoms from her husband to recognise the seriousness and import of these examinations. This only made her more frantic. She refused to go to the doctor again. She could not remain at home with those constant mementoes of her husband mocking her. She had to do something. She shut up her flat and went to live in a hotel. She withdrew from the entire world.

Withdrawal from the world of reality was, of course, the very worst thing that Helen R. could have done. She went from her cheerful apartment to live in a drab little hotel room, peopled with the ghostly obsessions of her own mind. She refused to follow her doctor's advice. She refused to work, and thus lost the counterbalance that comes from occupation. Her days were filled with pain, resentment, hate, and indecision; her nights were tortured by agonizing obsessions of her husband's infidelity, her own hopeless future, inner questionings, and introspective debates. She had always been a hard-working girl; she had lived morally; she had been charitable; she kept herself looking as young and attractive as she could. She had been sensitive to her husband's every wish, she had tried to be a good wife. And now, despite the fact that she had done everything that is prescribed in books on the good life, this shameful fate had overtaken her. Her friends shook their heads. Helen was in the throes of a nervous breakdown.

Dr. R. returned from abroad prepared to give an enthusiastic report of his trip. He had discounted the fact that he had received no mail from his wife for some weeks, and laid the blame on the eccentricities of Continental postal services rather than on his wife's remissness. He had received no answer to his telegram announcing his arrival, but then it did not really require an answer. His wife was a frugal business woman, and no doubt wanted to save the cost of a foreign telegram. He was sure she would meet him at the train. As his train pulled into the platform he scanned the faces and handkerchief-waving figures for a sight of his wife. He could find her nowhere. Perhaps she was waiting at the Customs. It would be sensible to avoid the crowd and greet him with a kiss under the big "R" of the Customs desk. But his wife was nowhere to be found.

You can imagine Dr. R.'s astonishment at finding his flat shut up, his wife not in her shop. When he finally discovered her in the hotel she was hardly recognisable. Her trim figure, her formerly cheerful face, her bright brown eyes were gone. He saw before him a haggard, unkempt, tearful, distracted, and almost incoherent woman who had lost hope and "face".

The cure of this case was not simple. Dr. R. fortunately was able to prove his absolute fidelity, because he had been accompanied on his entire trip by an older colleague who assured Helen R. that her husband had behaved himself in an exemplary fashion. This older colleague offered to face Mrs.

Brent (whose name, of course, is fictitious) with the facts, but Helen steadfastly refused to divulge her visitor's name or address. Gradually, under treatment, Helen's faith in her husband was restored, and her own face saved by the assurance that it had never been injured. But her moral code had to be changed. She was warned that there are in the world a great many neurotic women who achieve an insane sense of power by making trouble and carrying tales. With a husband as much in the public eye as Dr. R. she must be prepared to hear such stories from time to time. And so in time, with the constant repetition of assurances, she returned to her flat and began her life anew, with the added realisation that her husband, in his patient co-operation with the psychiatrist, had given unmistakable evidence of his love and devotion to her.

The case is illustrative, because it demonstrates how a critical situation may arise without the least warning; how even a well-adjusted individual may be called upon to "save face" under unusual circumstances; how a person who would have a reputation of being "100 per cent normal" may in such a critical situation show exactly the same symptoms that an individual with a long neurotic history would exhibit under similar circumstances; and finally, the fallacy of basing one's sense of "face" on a rigid moral code, upon a single ideal, upon a single technique of life.

HOMOSEXUAL BREAKDOWN

The case of Roland D. typifies the homosexual neurosis. Here a boy, unprepared to assume the normal sexual responsibilities of adult life, meets a confirmed homosexual who seduces him. Afraid of becoming involved in a homosexual life, Roland has a nervous breakdown. Psychological clarification brings him the peace and enjoyment of a normal heterosexual marriage.

So much misconception exists about homesexuality that we must include a case of homosexual breakdown in this chapter of erotic tragedies. The prevailing notion is that homosexuality is a congenital disease, due to a failure of proper sexual development before the individual's birth. The common belief is that both men and women with seemingly normal bodies exhibit the phenomenon of love for members of their own sex, because some pre-natal influence has warped their psycho-sexual point of view. This mistaken idea is responsible for a great deal of mischief in the history of the world. The belief that homosexuality is a moral vice, and, as such, deserving the condemnation and punishment of society is another popular fallacy. Misconception and misinformation about the nature of homosexuality have resulted in the widespread belief that homosexuality is an incurable perversion, a sort of moral leprosy. Any homosexual individual suffers the hate, the suspicion, and the ridicule of a society whose notions of this condition are fallacious, and which is often uncompromisingly hostile to him. In most countries the practice of homosexuality is still considered felonious, and the danger, therefore, that the affected individual will be subject to blackmail from unscrupulous individuals who understand how important it is for the homosexual to keep " face " publicly, is always present.

Let us say from the very outset that homosexuality is neither a congenital disease nor a moral vice. *Homosexuality is one symptom of a sexual neurosis.* It is not based on any pre-natal or congenital factor. It is not inherited. The homosexual neurosis, in the case of men, is based on the unconscious fear of the responsibility of adult sexual activity. Such qualms may include not only the fear of sexual contact with the female, but also the fear of sexual impotence, the fear of fatherhood, or the fear of being betrayed by the sexual mate. Like all other neuroses, it is an acquired strategy of life, and is based on factors conditioning childhood. In the case of women, Lesbianism (as female homosexuality is commonly called) is based on a similar fear of sexual relations, except that in the case of women, homosexuality is usually the symptom of a deep-lying masculine protest. Here the fear is bound up with the alleged sociological inferiority of woman that is taught us by law, tradition, custom, and even school books, in our patriarchal civilisation. The homosexual woman unconsciously believes that in submitting to the sexual embrace of the male she will actually be subjugated and robbed of her individuality and personality. This unconscious fear of sexual enslavement causes her to avoid all contact with the male, and to find love in the less dangerous arena of sexual contact with members of her own sex. In some cases, again, female homosexuality is due to the inhibiting influences of old wives' tales about the dangers of childbirth, or to the fear of the pains of childbirth.

Homosexuality, in either sex, is an unconscious " face-saving " technique based on false emotional patterns of fear which are laid down in early childhood. The homosexual neurosis is not inborn, but is acquired from the emotional reactions of the child to its parents. Like any other fallacious technique of life, homosexuality, can be cured by psychological analysis and re-education, notwithstanding all the wish-thinking of confirmed homosexuals to the contrary. We should like to say at this point that any individual who finds homosexuality an intolerable neurosis, and wants to become heterosexual, can be cured, no matter how long, or how intensely he has carried on his homosexual strategy.

As we pointed out in a previous case, the maintenance of one's sexual virility is one of the basic conditions of " face ". Individuals, therefore, who feel themselves "queer" or different in their sexual interests and activities, are frequently compelled to have a nervous breakdown, lest their dread secret be discovered. In many cases such individuals, because of our prevailing tradition of furtive secrecy in all matters of sex, cannot communicate their difficulties to anyone. They do not know where to look for guidance or help in their quandary. It is hoped that any reader who has tortured himself with such a secret for years will realise in reading these pages that any reputable psychiatrist will understand his problem, and lend him a sympathetic ear. The fear of the discovery of one's homosexual interest, the fear of the lonely old age that follows a career of homosexuality, the fear of loss of "face" in the eyes of one's family, friends, club, business, or social associates lays every homosexual and every potential homosexual especially open to the critical situations in which a nervous breakdown seems the only way out.

Just such an imminent loss of face occurred in the case of Roland D., the son of a doctor. Roland was the youngest son of a family of six children. An older brother dominated him during the early years of his life, and compelled him to submit to numerous homosexual indignities when he was only a young child. Roland's mother was not nearly as much interested in him as she was in his older brother. Roland's father, on the other hand, lavished his deepest affection on his youngest child, and wanted him to be either a doctor or an artist. No effort was spared to give him every artistic opportunity for development. Dr. D. was both mother and father to his son, as Mrs. D. was a cold, neurotic woman who had borne her children under protest, and had alienated most of the family with the exception of her first-born son who was her spoiled darling.

When Roland was eighteen, he was still in the midst of his storm and stress period of adolescence. He had become an elegant, æsthetically inclined, over-sensitive young man who laughed a great deal to hide his fear of his older brother. He was much sought after at social gatherings because of his musical and mimetic abilities, and was greatly liked by older people for his fine manners and graciousness. On Roland's nineteenth birthday his older brother was killed suddenly in an automobile accident. The older brother had always done the "regular" thing, played football at the university, gone into business, served in France as a Captain in the Artillery, and had got married. Roland had been perfectly willing to relinquish to his older brother the prerogatives of being "the man in the house". Suddenly the entire load of masculinity was thrown on his shoulders.

Roland always wanted to be an actor, but this career was very much frowned upon by all members of his family. His father was mildly disappointed that the boy did not enter medicine, but his mother actively and emphatically disapproved of a stage career. The family life was very close. Roland loved his sisters deeply, and lost no opportunity to visit them and their children. He was always in demand at parties because he could be counted upon to keep the company roaring with laughter. But despite the fact that Roland danced beautifully, was a thoughtful and considerate cavalier to the older ladies, he had no immediate interest in women. There had been two abortive love affairs while he was at college, but his mother had frowned on both girls, and Roland was so devoted to his family that he would never hurt them by marrying anyone who could not be brought into the intimate family circle.

After coming down from the university, Roland went into the theatre with all his heart and soul. He found the actors more interesting than the actresses. With several of them he had felt a strong emotional bond that had never been awakened in him by any girl. He liked to go out, it is true, with girls, even to make love to them in a superficial way, but he could not bring himself to have a serious love affair with anyone. With these young actors it was different. They seemed to speak his language. They had the same fine sensibilities that he had developed They did not run after women. They were " different ".

Roland was now twenty-eight years old. People were beginning to talk about him. He was being asked constantly why he did not marry, why he went around only with " queer " men. Women who liked him for his charm and good looks, but who found him uninterested in any sexual dalliance, began to speak of him as a homosexual. Roland was annoyed at first by these imputations, and then depressed. He was afraid there was something wrong with him because he could not develop a desire for any girl. He did not know with whom he could speak about these matters. He instinctively feared to discuss his sexual life with his father, because his father, too, had joined the insistent contingent of those who wanted him to marry.

Then something happened which changed Roland's entire life. He met an older actor who held an important position in the world of the theatre. This actor, whom we shall call Mr. Blake, seemed to take a great interest in Roland. He took him around to clubs, to which Roland had previously had had no *entrée*. He gave Roland instructions in acting and directing, and put him in touch with the most influential producers. Little by little Roland sensed that Mr. Blake had more than a mere fatherly interest in him. He often went to see Mr. Blake in his exotic studio. And one night when Roland had come to Blake's studio after a late party he invited him to spend the night. " There's no sense in your driving out to the suburbs at this hour! " he had pleaded. Roland stayed, and Blake after a long recitation of his own personal conversion to homosexuality, induced Roland to submit to his sexual embraces. Blake told Roland how he had struggled for years to find an interest in women. He repeated the well-known fallacies about the congenital nature of homosexuality. He convinced Roland that his happiness could come only if he dedicated himself to a life of sexual inversion.

Roland was confused. On the one hand he realised the greater wisdom and experience of Blake. Compared to this man he was an unsophisticated child. In their relations he experienced a thrill that had never come to him from any woman he had ever known. At the same time he realised that he would be ostracised from his family if it became known that he was a homosexual. He had dimly recognised that he was " different " from other men, and had long sought guidance on the matter. But the books he had read only confused him the more. And now this older man was filling his mind with ideas that were at one and the same time repulsive and alluring to him. Blake became more and more possessive and jealous and Roland recognised the fact that the relation was an unwholesome one. He seemed hypnotised by the man's suave explanations. Blake gave him books and more books to read. Suddenly Roland recognised the full import of his relationship with Blake. He was becoming a homosexual! To be a homosexual meant the complete loss of his family. He remembered only too well hearing his father say, " I'd rather have a son of mine dead than have him a sexual pervert! "

Roland became miserable and depressed. He

wanted to be a normal man. He wanted to marry and have children and grow into a responsible human being. Blake kept poisoning his mind, dangling the irresponsible allurements of a homosexual life before his eyes. Roland felt that success in his profession must not be bought at the expense of losing the respect of his family. The enormity of his sexual relationship with Blake began to oppress him. There seemed no solution to the problem.

All he could do was to think about the nights that he had spent with Blake. He found himself looking at men as he passed them on the street and sensing a sexual thrill when a good-looking man touched him. He felt that he had condemned himself irrevocably to a career of homosexuality. The fear of being discovered agonised him. His family began to criticise his actions; he became slovenly and disinterested. He slept late, sometimes remaining at home for days, making no progress in his stage career. At night he would go to Blake's as if drawn by an invisible magnet. Then he would return home in the morning, tired, disgusted, and despondent. He could not overcome his indecision. Which way should he go? Should he lose " face " with the family and win fame in the theatre at the price of homosexuality, or should he renounce Blake and try to get married, although Blake had often told him he would be unhappy in marriage? Finally, his habits became so bad, he lost so much weight, he became so preoccupied and distracted, that his father sent him to me for a consultation. Roland had given up all hope. He was in a blue funk, totally discouraged, totally confused, totally unfit to solve the problem of his nervous breakdown.

Let us examine the factors in this case. The background: a youngest and spoiled child, given an inferiority complex by a dominant and aggressive brother, and an unthinking, cold-hearted, undemonstrative mother. This boy learned to find love and help only from his father, and never knew what it was to have kindness and sympathy from a woman. Naturally, in later life, he turned toward males to find love, appreciation and the demonstration of affection. At the same time the exceptionally close family life gave him a limited arena in which to find " face " and a full sense of values. The approval of his closely-knit family was much more important than the approval of the outside world. For the first years of his life he developed æsthetically, as a means of gaining his father's affection, leaving all more " masculine " forms of training to his brother. Then suddenly he had to assume the whole burden of the masculinity of the family when his brother died. For this he felt unprepared. He drifted, therefore, into the theatre, where he could at least gain a subjective sense of superiority by acting the rôle, rather than being a man and assuming the objective responsibilities of masculinity.

The environment of the theatre threw him into contact with other neurotic individuals who were running away from reality, and he found comfort in their company. While the heterosexual ideals of his family were uppermost in his mind, he had unconsciously avoided their responsibilities by remaining a " playboy " all his life. Then the affair with Blake brought him to the realisation that he was " different " and he felt destined and dedicated to a life of homosexuality. This misconception made him suddenly fear that he would be compelled to relinquish the affection and " face " demanded by his family, particularly his father. The nervous breakdown, therefore, unmasks itself as an attempt to camouflage the bitter truth, that he was a homosexual (as Blake had deluded him into accepting), while his multiplex physical symptoms served to re-enlist the sympathies of his doctor father, as in his childhood when he had turned to him for love, sympathy and the assuaging of every little pain.

The cure of the case consisted in demonstrating the utter fallacy of Blake's teachings, and the inculcation into Roland of the belief that he could be just as normal as any other man, despite his bad training. The rôle of the vicious conditioning factors, from his older brother's forcing him into a homosexual relation to Blake's luring him into the same type of relation, was made clear to him. The basic emotional error of his life, that all women were like his neurotic mother, cold, calculating, unsympathetic, and that unconsciously he had expected similar undemonstrativeness from other women, was pointed out. He was taught to look at women on the street, instead of unconsciously allowing his gaze to fasten on men.

The rôle of his symptoms as an attention-getting device was similarly demonstrated. He was told that he did not have to embark on a career of sexual relations with women immediately, but that his first job was to make friends of women. He was helped over the first steps by being taken out of the environment of his family (where everyone had been commenting disparagingly on his changed attitude and different looks), and was urged to build up a new social milieu among strangers. He began looking out for other people instead of looking out only for himself. He organized a marionette theatre for the children of a settlement house as a means of getting his thoughts off his own body and his own symptoms. This marionette theatre brought him considerable fame, and it became a vogue. Everyone wanted him to give marionette performances for their children. In this way he came into contact with many fine sympathetic women, and finally met a young artist who was greatly interested in the theatre, and married her. They work together now, are completely happy sexually, and all Roland's homosexual desires and activities are entirely gone.

Roland writes, "These men who think they are women and try to act like women, are really not feminine . . . they are like a cheap actor's impersonation of femininity. The whole thing is artificial, and when you are given objective eyes to see it with, it all seems like a very shoddy parade. I say that normality is the easiest and most natural way to live. That's why it's normal. As for me, the whole sorry story of my wanderings through the maze of sex is like a bad, half-forgotten nightmare now. I'm so busy with my work for the theatre, and so happy in the love of my wife, that I have no time even to think of it any more. But I do believe the medical profession should actively spread the truth about homosexuality and offer its services to those who are going through the mental travail that I have experienced during my breakdown. It seems much more important to me that all these young men be saved than that millions be spent in research on the obscure diseases of the Hottentots."

And with this we end the chapter of the nervous breakdowns based on sexual themes. If your nervous breakdown has been conditioned by sexual misinformation and miseducation, the successful outcome of this wide range of cases should give you courage. What others have done, you, too, can accomplish. Others have been through the same torture and agony, and have recovered their peace of mind. You, too, can get well.

CHAPTER FIVE

OF CASES AND CURES—PART III

Economic Breakdown: *The case of Jack M., a former American millionaire, who amassed a fabulous fortune to compensate for his inferiority complex. The sudden loss of his money robs him of his self-esteem. A nervous breakdown temporarily saves him from the consequences of his folly, until psychological insight enables him to make a fresh start in life.*—National Economic Breakdown—Reactions Toward Depression—Emergency Exits from Reality—The Martyr Complex—After the Depression, What?—Facing the Music—Making the Most of Adversity—Family Breakdown: *The case of the D. family, illustrates the havoc caused by a too close relationship between mother and son. This case not only shows the vicious influence of in-laws and spiritualism, but also the curative power of music and love.*—Miscellaneous Breakdowns.

ECONOMIC BREAKDOWN

The case of Jack M., a former American millionaire, who amassed a fabulous fortune to compensate for his inferiority complex. The sudden loss of his money robs him of his self-esteem. A nervous breakdown temporarily saves him from the consequences of his folly, until psychological insight enables him to make a new start in life.

IN our civilisation the worth of a man is usually measured by the size of his bank account. Any individual suffering from an inferiority complex is likely to succumb to this international fallacy, and attempt to gain security by aggressively amassing a fortune. But in no country is the possession of money so commonly the chief fiction of power as in the United States. The legion of American men and women who base their sense of " face " on money and its implied power supplies the recruits to the haggard army of neurotics, whose members are forced to have nervous breakdowns simply because they have lost their money.

When we speak of economic causes for nervous breakdown, we must distinguish between two types. The first type is characteristic of this age and time. In the machine age we see the phenomenon of a whole society sick because of its over-valuation and misuse of money. This handbook is no place to discuss the philosophy of economics, yet it must be apparent to every intelligent reader that our whole society is affected with a mental disorder, whose symptoms alternate between periods of hypo-manic " business booms " and phases of melancholic " business depression ". When the nations are sick it is inevitable that thousands of citizens will be sacrificed on the altar of national madness. During the early years of American history, as during the period of prosperity and industrial development in England, it was taught that hard work and perseverance would make any man rich and respected. While there were virgin fields to exploit this philosophy worked very well. Individuals failed and had nervous breakdowns because they could not stand the strain of a competitive society, but in the majority of instances the rule applied and held good.

To-day, however, we must face the facts of the disappearance of virgin fields of exploitation, and the shrinkage of pioneer areas. We can no longer be blind to the spectre of over-production for profit, nor deny the stalking ghosts and wraiths of under-consumption. Throughout the world millions starve in the face of plenty; machines rust while willing hands remain idle, and thousands of healthy men with the desire to work and to produce are kept unemployed and despondent so that a few others can barely make a living wage. The old fiction of "rugged individualism" has been exploded, and thousands of victims stand helpless, deprived of their natural birthright, the right to work and win "face" and esteem by their labour. They have nervous breakdowns because they have been compelled to become dependent on public charity for support, and the dole they receive signifies to them a "loss of face". They can no longer look their wives, children, and neighbours in the face.

We have no recourse but to take care of them and their dependents as public charges. It is the staggering price that must be paid for national madness. The insanity of current economic philosophies must be apparent to anyone who knows the sad facts. We see the pitiful results of economic " muddling through " on all sides. Moral and physical degradation beset the unfortunate victims of our present economic depression as never before. If we saw an individual going through a performance comparable to such behaviour, we would commit him to an insane asylum for a period of observation! Suppose a man, on Wednesday, talked volubly of his supersalesmanship, his unbounded enthusiasm, his faith in the eternal rightness of things, and acted as if he were supremely indifferent to anyone's opinion of him. Suppose this same man were to awake on Thursday, his confidence shattered, his boasts turned to whining complaints, his enthusiasms transformed over night into blackest despair, his cock-sureness become abject humility. We would certainly remove such a man to a mental hospital and put a label of " manic-depressive psychosis " at the foot of his bed, and restrain him forcibly from injuring himself or others.

Psychiatrists are not prophets in their own countries and therefore such therapy cannot be applied to whole nations. The manic-depressive nation, like the manic-depressive individual, will not listen to reason while things are going well, and when things go badly it wants a narcotic (in our case the spiritual lollypop called prosperity), not commonsense advice on how to change its childish ways. We must, therefore, wait either until the fantastic absurdity of our present system produces such terrifying consequences that the very logic of reality will compel a change, or until our entire civilisation will follow the way of past civilisations, and destroy itself and us. Until this happens those who are the victims of the system must become workers for national and international sanity.

The type of nervous breakdown which has an economic and critical situation as a basis concerns us more directly in this handbook of help and self-help. The case of Jack M. is characteristic. At the age of ten, Jack came to the United States, an immigrant boy from Russia. He had seen his elder brothers slaughtered before his eyes by drunken Cossacks in a pogrom. Jack M. was small, Jewish, clumsy and uncouth, but he was fired by an aggressive ambition to compensate for the precarious existence of his youth, by making a fortune in the promised land. He learned quickly because adversity had sharpened his wits. He worked by day and studied at night. He had spent his childhood in the cramped and dank quarters of a ghetto, and he compensated by acquiring a knowledge of real estate values. He became a lawyer, and combined both sets of special knowledge, so that at the age of forty Jack M. was a successful man. He had married and was the father of three children. Part of his ambition was to watch his children grow up to be ladies and gentlemen. He wanted them to know nothing of the hardships which he had endured. " Let them have the best educations, marry well and carry on the tradition of my rise to power," he said. At the age of forty-five, thanks to his native shrewdness and the unlimited possibilities of a manic period of national inflation, Jack M. was a millionaire, His wife wore the most expensive furs, each child had his own motor car, his daughter had been educated at the finest finishing school, and his sons were at the most famous universities.

Jack was a magician in the legerdemain of interlocking directorships, "holding" companies, "watered" stocks. He had always been honest, as far as one can be honest in the service of Mammon, by "honestly" manipulating the stock market, buying on margin here, selling short there. His good wife, a girl of sound peasant stock, had been frankly alarmed by the piling up of his enormous wealth, and had begged Jack to retire and enjoy his millions. But Jack was in the manic phase. He spent his money lavishly. He bought his way into the highest places, and came back to his wife, chuckling like a small boy, to tell her how this or the other member of the Four Hundred had come to him for a favour. He was drunk with the power of his money, and he had no basis for his self-esteem other than his vast financial holdings.

And then, on his fifty-first birthday, he awoke, with his doctor anxiously feeling his pulse, telling him that he had angina pectoris, a dangerous heart disease, and his secretary telling him that he was a ruined man. His financial balloon had been pricked by the needle of the depression. It lay on the ground a shrivelled bag of deflated hopes. Jack M. had taken many rebuffs in his life, but he could not withstand this onslaught of destiny. He seemed aged and haggard. He had lost a small fortune once before, and had suffered a minor mental depression in consequence, but he had remade his " pile " without difficulty, and as soon as he had money in the bank again, his good spirits had returned. But that was when he was but thirty-eight years old, healthy, full of confidence and ambition. Now, for the first time in many years, he was in a state of panic. Pictures of the pogrom which he had witnessed as a child of five kept recurring to him. He felt remorseful for not having been more charitable, although he had never been known to deny any charity worker a contribution for a worthy cause. Now he was the object of charity. It put him back forty-five years, to the misery of a Russian ghetto beyond the pale.

It ruined him both mentally and financially. He could not even pay his doctor's bills. Creditors besieged him. Hundreds of small investors who had lost their life's savings, because they had played gullible mercenaries to his over-confident rôle of " the Mussolini of real estate ", clamoured for retribution. In his fitful slumber he could hear their shrill voices, their imprecations and their wails. He refused to see any of his old friends. His body seemed racked with intolerable pains. He cursed his business associates for " selling him out ". He feared death and became a bed-ridden tyrant. Physical symptoms kept his wife at his bedside night and day. He threatened suicide. The entire family had to take turns in restraining him from jumping out of his window.

This was the course of his nervous breakdown. When everyone had deserted him, his wife stood by his side and ministered to his eccentric, often insane demands. Finally, she, too, could stand the strain of his tyranny no more. The physician, who had looked after Jack's bodily health for many years, assured me that there was no organic basis for the variety and intensity of his symptoms. Jack would not listen to his physician's advice, and refused to call a psychiatrist in consultation. Enough of his megalomania remained to make the admission of mental defeat untenable. His remaining vestige of " face " could not brook such intervention in his plight. This is a difficult point with many individuals who suffer a nervous breakdown. They are so obsessed with the physical nature of their symptoms, that they refuse to consult those who understand that symptoms are but the broadcasting of mental despair, and are best trained to help them to recover their mental equilibrium. Jack had lost his " face " financially. However, he maintained, to the last his belief in his own ability to help himself out of the abyss into which he had plunged.

The case, therefore, was treated indirectly by his

doctor and his wife, under my guidance. Jack was removed to a little camp in the Adirondacks which had not yet been attached by his creditors. His wife, the doctor, and one son went to live with him. He was kept on a strict regime of rest for a period of weeks. During the heyday of his prosperity Jack had developed a great liking for good music, and a little gramophone and a good collection of records helped to soothe him. Then a regular routine of easy exercise was instituted. After a while he emulated the great failure of Doorn, and chopped wood regularly in the mornings. Gradually, under the fostering influence of his psychologically trained doctor and his sensible wife, Jack recovered some semblance of his mental equanimity and physical peace. After three months he returned to the city considerably restored. A course in psychological readings had reconciled him to psychiatric treatment, especially when his physician told him that he owed his restoration to health to my indirect regimen.

In the treatment of any nervous breakdown we must use all existing personality assets as a lever. Here was a man who was not essentially bad or malicious. Misguided, over-ambitious, vain, over-aggressive, he certainly was, but he was neither morally corrupt, nor basically anti-social. The treatment must give the patient an opportunity to regain his " face ". The first thing was to help him make restitution. Then he was put to the task of preparing legislation which would inhibit unscrupulous or over-ambitious financiers from " putting over " such schemes of personal aggrandisement as his own.

To-day, Jack M. is soberly at work. His yacht, his magnificent penthouse, his three limousines, his extensive real estate holdings are gone. He lives in a modest apartment, works ten hours a day, rides in the subway and greets his friends with a firm handshake. He is using his knowledge to improve the housing conditions of the poor. He is not afraid of death or heart disease. He looks hopefully to the future as to the quiet epilogue of a mad play. He is a changed man.

NATIONAL ECONOMIC BREAKDOWN

Jack M.'s case is so characteristic of what is happening in the whole world to-day that in analysing its dynamics we may simultaneously analyse the current depression. Neurotic techniques are human. Men who control national destinies are human. It is inevitable that the fallacious techniques of fallible human beings should creep into our national attitudes and conduct. Let us see how far we can make the analogy that the United States, or, for that matter, most of the industrialised nations of the world, to-day act like a neurotic patient with a tendency to cyclothymia, or manic-depressive insanity, fit the facts.

Nations react to calamity exactly as individuals.

Any national disaster (analogous to the critical situation of the individual pattern of conduct) is likely to produce national reactions comparable to those generated by the breakdown of a romantic life-formula in an individual confronted with his first frustration by reality. The sole difference that might logically be expected is the difference in the degree and variety of the symptoms. The child who must relinquish his belief in Santa Claus makes one specific, individual and characteristic neurotic response. The nation, being an aggregation of such individuals, is more likely to display the entire galaxy of neurotic devices simultaneously and in every degree of intensity.

From the point of view of human reactions, the current depression signalises a breakdown of the most respected clichés of American thought. The average American is imbued with an uncritical belief in the eternal rightness of all things American. No American army has ever been bested in any important encounter. Big Business, with all that the phrase implies, has always been considered as right as God and the Constitution. American independence, self-sufficiency, and isolation have never been questioned, while American speed, sports, technical developments, advertisements, and our scale of living in general, have become the standards of the world.

The depression has cast grave doubts on the validity of many of these beliefs, and proved others to be utterly incredible and unreliable. In the case of Jack M. it was his fundamental belief, that shrewdness and foresight were the only necessary qualifications for complete success, that was exploded. For the first time in history, healthy Americans of native stock are starving in the midst of plenty. The vaunted " splendid isolation " and the time-honoured detachment of American diplomacy have become untenable principles. Big Business, the last of the American idols to expose its clay feet, has been unmasked as a fraud and a delusion. Men who have never questioned the belief that hard work, honesty, and the investment of one's savings in " sound " stocks and bonds would eventually guarantee a comfortable security, are wearily pounding the streets in search of jobs. Others who have retained their jobs have developed a panicky slave-morality towards their employers. And to cap the climax, the luxuries and comforts of American living, which have become an almost universal tradition, have completely collapsed. The never-before-questioned rightness of unrestrained competitive individualism has proved itself a fatal boomerang. The great American myth has been exploded.

The effect of this collapse on the average American man and woman has been almost identical with the collapse of a romantic notion in the life plan of a blustering, over-aggressive adolescent. The bewildered child who learns for the first time that Easter bunnies do not lay Easter eggs and that the stork does not bring babies, is the psychological model of the behaviour of the average American in the current depression. The adolescent who discovers that the God to whom he has been praying all his life is not universally accredited, or the university graduate who discovers in his first month of business that a degree from his university is not a *carte blanche* to commercial success, exhibits the same devastating doubt and discouragement that the psychiatrist finds in the average present-day American. Perhaps the best parallel of all is to be found in the case of the romantic youth who falls in love with the girl of his dreams. He marries her amid a fanfare of trumpets and a barrage of rice and old shoes in the most acceptable and traditional fashion, only to find after a brief honeymoon that his wife cannot budget the family accounts, cannot cook a simple meal, demands an excess of romantic affection, and is a cry-baby into the bargain.

REACTIONS TOWARD DEPRESSION

When a romantically adolescent individual is confronted with an unpleasant reality, there are ten neurotic courses open to him—and one normal one. Needless to say, it is the normal course alone that can cure the breakdown. In the neurotic categories he may do the following:

1. Admit his failure, but continue in his old

habits and beliefs on the theory that his present failure is an exception to the rule of his former successes. Such an individual usually redoubles his efforts in the same fallacious manner as before, hopeful to the end that his unique private logic will be vindicated. He may refuse to admit the existence of the difficulty and continue to reiterate his time-worn mottoes and ideas in the manner of the much maligned ostrich.

2. He may embark upon a career of hectic hedonism and attempt to find solace in the mad pursuit of pleasures and diversions. This strategy follows on the unconscious admission of complete defeat and the equally unconscious breakdown of all hope for the future.

3. He may seek supernatural aid to help him out of his difficulties.

4. He may refuse to accept his own responsibility for his failure and search for a scapegoat on whose unwilling back he may unload his own shortcomings. In the case of Jack M. his heart was the scapegoat.

5. He may become suddenly panic-stricken, forget his sense of proportion, and try to commit suicide.

6. He may develop a martyr complex, and indulge himself in an orgy of self-pity, self-castigation, and self-humiliation. Remorse and penance are variations of this complex. This mechanism is obvious in Jack's remorse at having wrecked the

lives of depositors, his shame at not having contributed more to charity.

7. He may attempt to propitiate the unfriendly fates by minor acts of sacrifice, without any true insight into the nature of his situation.

8. He may submit meekly to the insults of destiny, because he is so burdened with a guilt complex derived from an authoritarian education that he knows no other course.

9. He may develop a paranoid hatred for the particular situation he holds accountable for his misfortunes, and spend his energy in futile fuming, cursing, and gnashing of teeth, without actually doing anything about it.

10. He may set up a side show in which his frantic activity seems to distract the attention of the onlooker from his own plight. Here he may bolster his self-esteem by recounting the glories of his past and pointing to the greater difficulties of his neighbours. Jack's bedside tyranny was an attempt of this kind. Having lost everything, he wanted to make certain that he was still the master of his household.

And finally, in the category of mature reactions, he may study his failure objectively, understand the factors that led to his débâcle, and begin his training toward the prevention of similar disasters in the future. Needless to say this latter course is the only one consistent with future success, sanity, and happiness.

In the first category of neurotic responses we find " 100 percenters " who cannot admit that the economic depression is anything out of the ordinary. Their thought processes are so benumbed by old " bromides " that it is practically impossible for them to conceive an American failure. Their only course is to redouble their efforts in the good old direction toward national snobbery and the deification of individualism. They continue to raise the tariff walls and avert their glances from starving miners, musicians, engineers, and teachers. " Prosperity ", one of the great American myths, is " just around the corner " for them. The depression is only a bad dream. " America always comes out on top," they say. " We've had depressions before and we always came out of them. Just let things take their natural course." This philosophy seldom emanates from those who are vitally touched by the untoward effects of depression. It comes from well-fed men and women entrenched in relatively strong positions. They can afford to minimise the depression. They have their incomes, roofs over their heads, and usually motor cars in their garages.

EMERGENCY EXITS FROM REALITY

In the second category, however, we find that discouragement has appeared and a definitely neurotic pattern of life is assumed. The depression is admitted in all its drab horror, and an attitude of complete hopelessness pervades the individual's outlook on the future. Men and women of this group act as if they were dancing on the rim of an active and grumbling volcano. The *débâcle* may come at any time. Therefore seize the day and make merry, for to-morrow you are likely to find yourself in the workhouse, or begging on the streets. The artificial narcosis of alcohol, morphine, night clubs, and of sexual excesses offers immediate surcease from the tragic disillusion of the present. The immediate pleasure of intoxication is not only a flight from reality: it becomes the ultimate goal of existence for men and women in this category. As in the first category, this mechanism of escape has obviously dangerous characteristics. We may expect an increase in drunkenness, drug addiction, jazz-mania, and sexual delinquency as a consequence of this type of reaction, not only for the duration of the depression, but also for a long time after it has passed.

The third type of neurotic response is closely associated with the second. In this instance we find grown men and women, many of whom have had the advantage of good education, men and women who have been successful during the boom days, in frantic search for new magical formulae, because their sense of humour has been completely undermined by the failure of their erstwhile magic. The hankering for magic is deeply rooted in the human breast. And when the neurotic loses confidence in the magic of the dollar he is very likely to seek the magic of the astrologer, the numerologist, the phrenologist, the fortune-teller, the mystic, the spiritualist, and the faith-healer. Unbelievably large sums are spent in the United States every year for the spurious advice of these pseudo-scientific gentry. Bank presidents who have lost their inner fortitude repress their critical faculties, and sit like little children listening to the babble of suave oracles who know nothing of economics but a great deal about the gullibility of men. There is no more distressing spectacle than this sorry picture of ignorance, timidity, superstition, and spinelessness. There will be no depression for the astrologers and numerologists as long as " Big Business " executives consult witches and wizards instead of text-books on economics, history, political science, sociology, and modern psychology for counsel.

In the fourth category of neurotic reactions to the depression, we find the ancient and honourable cult of devil-chasing and scapegoat-baiting enthroned in all its pristine pomp. During the Middle Ages, when men believed fervently in the Devil, it was a relatively simple matter to blame Satan for all human shortcomings and every miscarriage of human plans and desires. When Spain was going through its great economic depression in the fifteenth century, the Jews were the scapegoat, and their expulsion became an act of highest piety. Hitlerite Germany, having, like the Bourbons, learned nothing and forgotten nothing from history, follows the Spanish custom to-day. The tendency to find a scapegoat for our failure is almost as deeply ingrained in our unconscious minds as the desire for magical panaceas. And, just as we might have expected in a country whose most pious beliefs have been shattered, we find the sport of devil-chasing in the United States centred in the mass hysteria of Bolshevik-baiting. Those terrible Russians! They are responsible for all our misery and misfortune. The tragi-comic spectacle of New York City's police beating up defiant young Communists with a yearning for martyrdom, as well as the ultimate clowning of Congressional investigations of Communist activities, are eloquent evidence of the popularity of the scapegoat-finding technique of meeting the realities of the depression.

The fifth group of reactions is among the most tragic of those that have developed in the present situation. These are the suicides. The tragedy in the suicide lies not so much in the actual loss of life, deplorable as this may be in itself, but in the tragic fallacy of the underlying technique of life. One of the most revered myths in America is the fiction that money is power. Probably more worshippers are to be found at the shrine of Mammon in this country than in any other in the world. Even those who do not worship directly before the golden calf often believe implicitly in the power of American bankers and money to control the destinies of the world and, indirectly, to keep the American worker's standard of living the highest in the world.

It is not surprising, therefore, that so many Americans have devoted themselves whole-heartedly and with unique singleness of purpose to the acquisition of money. The great majority of Americans probably consider a fat bank account synonymous with happiness. The sudden deflation of these artificial standards of happiness has left the deluded and narrow-minded devotees of money in desperate straits. Financial deflation spells mental bankruptcy for them. Suicide appears as the only emergency exit to those who have completely lost their courage and who have never developed more than one technique of life. Those who are left behind are forced to bear the additional burdens of the suicide's demise, plus the accrued heartache of a sense of guilt for the implied responsibility of his failure.

THE MARTYR COMPLEX

In the sixth category we find one of the commonest neurotic reactions that has developed since the Stock Market crash of 1929: a spurious martyr complex. Visitors who came to America from harassed Central European countries, where the populations have suffered and faced depression far more intense than any we have ever known in the United States, are amazed at the American talk about depression. This neurotic reaction has definitely become the vogue. Certainly it has become the commonest excuse for every conceivable asocial act, from the sweating of employees to the enforced exaction of contributions from already overburdened and underpaid workers. A psychological pall has settled over the country. In sections where business has not been abnormally affected, the extension of the pessimistic bleatings of other sections has served to develop a veritable anxiety neurosis. The depression has disclosed the fact that the American nation, which has always prided itself on its good sportsmanship and on its ability to be a good loser, is actually a nation of panicky cry-babies. As a nation Americans are good sports when they are winning everything in sight. They have developed the delusion that they could never lose. Such delusions are psychologically disastrous. The depression has shown up the average American as a superstitious, socially mal-adjusted, politically naïve, economically unawakened, psychologically immature adolescent crying for the lost lollypop of prosperity, and pathetically incapable of doing anything fundamental or constructive about it.

In the seventh category fall those good-hearted Americans who listen to the appeals of the various emergency relief institutions and dig generously into their pockets to help the unemployed, at the same time remaining ignorant of the deeper implications of the present social cataclysm. These good people feel they have done their bit when they have contributed to their local charities, and allow the matter to end there. It is as if they propitiated the avenging furies with the small coin of charity, and then retreated into the fastnesses of their own little egos. Charity without insight is worse than useless. In this category of reactions we find the apotheosis of social *laissez-faire*.

In the eighth important classification we must put the unemployed, the university and technical school graduates who cannot get a job, and the workers who, despite willingness to work, can only find a partial occupation, or are compelled to do menial work instead of the technical work they are trained to do. The disintegrating effects of long periods of unemployment on the human psyche are not usually recognised outside the domain of psychiatrists, social workers, and relief agencies. Psychologically the most interesting phenomenon of our current difficulties is the extraordinary meekness and the unbelievable acquiescence and submission of the American workers out of a job. Just as the Army Intelligence Tests in the War taught America that it was a nation of morons, so the depression has taught it that it is a nation of masochists. The European worker out of a job usually demands political action. The unemployed American sits at home, listens to his radio if he has not been dispossessed of it, stands humbly in a bread line, applies apologetically to a social agency for relief and, if refused, submits to the most intolerable indignities. Slave morality has grown apace, and is found not only in the case of the panic-stricken jobholder who lives in terror lest he should lose his job, but even more so among the unemployed, who exhibit not the least trace of rebellion at their condition.

AFTER THE DEPRESSION, WHAT?

The mass masochism of the American worker out of a job is doubtless the product of our authoritarian education. Our schools place a premium on obedience and conformity rather than on independence of thought and judgment. If our workers had been taught to be moie resourceful, certain pernicious psychological effects of unemployment would have been considerably ameliorated. Just as this same authoritarian education, with its over-emphasis on "practical" matters has led to nervous breakdowns and neuroses among the well-to-do, who have experienced a compulsory spiritual bankruptcy when confronted with the reality of an existence without affluence (as was the case with Jack M.), so, among the workers, the identical one-sided education has effected a veritable mass neurosis of discouragement and despair. We are now just beginning to feel the effects of this spineless submission. The next twenty years, however, will show the terrific costs of our lack of social vision. Insane asylums and jails will be overflowing. The available mental hygiene facilities that were hopelessly inadequate in times of prosperity will be pathetically overcrowded in future years, when the children who are experiencing the devastating effects of the breakdown of morale in their parents of to-day will themselves have to face the problems of to-morrow. It requires no far-sighted prophet to picture the disintegration of these stunted minds and bodies ten, fifteen, and twenty years hence. Physical want and privation are the easily visible consequences of the depression. The effects of fear, of loss of self-confidence, of discouragement, of continued submission and masochism, are to be counted as even more serious consequences still. They are the liabilities which future generations will have to shoulder.

In the ninth category of reactions we may classify all those whom psychiatrists would consider more or less paranoid.[1] The depression-paranoiacs are incensed because they have been jolted out of their equanimity, and their chief reactions are hate and anger toward those who have not suffered so much from the depression, or toward those who seem, to the paranoiacs, responsible for their discomfiture. On the one hand we have the explosive Anarchists who believe that bombs are a solution to social problems, and on the other hand the fantastic monomaniacs who believe that the depression was ordered in the Soviet Councils. The search for panaceas is in the same category. There are large groups of Americans who believe that the return of three per cent beer,

[1] Paranoia is a psychosis, or form of insanity, which is characterised by a fixed delusional system, most frequently of persecution.

a bigger navy, or a subsidy for the farmers will magically lift the entire depression. Others feel that the wholesale deportation of all foreigners would accomplish the same result. Still others clamour for bimetallism, or a dictator. Preachers call on their flocks to return to the Golden Rule, and university professors pray for a return to the classics. They belong to the army of cranks, eccentrics, micro-paranoiacs seeking for magical formulae.

The tenth category of reactions comprises all those side-show activities designed to divert our attention from the gravity of the present social crisis. Men and women who regard the inflation period as a pleasant dream, and resign themselves to the present situation as if this were the ordinary expected course of events, belong in this group, as do their neighbours who exonerate the breakdown of American ideals and institutions by pointing, with questionable pride, to the world-wide demoralization of competitive individualism, adding the unspoken corollary, "Well, we are not so badly off. The poor Germans are in a worse plight!" The recounting of the past glories of American history likewise falls into this side-show category. The truth is that no matter how busy we are in our interest in the artificial importance of sports, prize-fighting, or the breakdown of other nations, we cannot hide the fact that we are, ourselves, confronted with a demoralizing bankruptcy, a complete invalidation of formerly unquestioned shibboleths.

FACING THE MUSIC

So much for the black side of the picture. There remains an important category of consequences and reactions that promises a " normalising tendency ". The depression has opened the eyes of many Americans, who in the past have been content to dismiss the matter of social responsibility with that pet phrase " the poor we have always with us ". It has demonstrated the fact that all unemployed men are not professional beggars, and it has shown all too clearly how utterly insecure the American worker is in his job, how dependent on the caprice of his employer. This widening of social horizons and this intensification of interest in the problems of other workers and other sections and types of Americans can be put down as one of the indubitable benefits of the depression. It required a nervous breakdown to teach Jack M. that knowledge of real estate values could be used to improve housing conditions of the poor just as easily as it could be utilised to make money for himself. This is the normal reaction of an individual who has come face to face with an insuperable obstacle, and analyses his failure to meet it objectively. In the present situation a great many Americans who formerly were content to let Uncle Sam take care of everything have realised their own social responsibility for the first time. If the deplorable depression has had no other effect, it is valuable in that it has stimulated these reactions.

Intelligent men and women who have studied our national plight recognise the breakdown of our culture and the insolvency of our national worship of unrestrained competitive individualism. It is apparent that the depression has affected those whose life work is one of service and social co-operation less than it has affected others whose objective has been the acquisition of wealth. It has proved, if it has done nothing else, that as a nation we have no idea of the valid use of leisure. It has piled up mountains of evidence indicating the importance of versatility, the need for personal resourcefulness, and the vital necessity of community social planning. Above all, the financial depression has stimulated in thousands of men and women who were formerly content to drift with the tide the desire to know more, to develop intellectual resources, to learn new techniques, with the result that the adult education movement has been greatly fostered and extended. Thousands of Americans, who would have considered the proposal to continue their studies after school or university as ludicrous, are now hard at their books again.

MAKING THE MOST OF ADVERSITY

The history of the human race is full of examples of the auspicious and beneficial affects of adversity. Our current depression is no exception to this rule. The human spirit develops best under pressure. It is true that the lame ducks we have allowed to grow up in our *laissez-faire* culture will suffer horribly under this adversity, and that those who are responsible and mature will have to assume their burdens, as in bygone days. But more and more men and women will find in the depression a stimulus to the expansion of mental horizons and the extension of human sympathies. The depression has taught us a lesson that our troglodyte ancestors learned early in the course of human evolution: the necessity of social co-operation.

The future is a matter of conjecture. If the depression lifts quickly no one will have learned much from it, just as Jack M. learned nothing from his first loss of fortune and his first miniature breakdown. As soon as the stock market begins to soar, the same old insane worship of Mammon will begin over again, the same number of suckers will be caught in the meshes of an aggressive, money-mad individualism. The same old bromides, clichés, mottoes, and shibboleths will be repeated as solemnly as ever before.

If it continues a great deal longer the toll of crime and insanity and the epidemic spread of neuroses, delinquency, suicide, generalised discouragement, and hopelessness may lead us to a social cataclysm—or to a new social order based on adult recognition of our social responsibilities. The smaller the world grows, the more apparent it becomes to every thinking man and woman that each individual is responsible for human welfare. For the present it would be well for every American to realise that there is no peculiar magic that rules over American institutions and ideals. It is not written in the book of destiny that we shall escape the fate of other lost civilisations who staked all on power and might and riches. We must face the insolvency of the past squarely and objectively, and begin to plan for a future based not on superstition, on magical mottoes, on *laissez-faire* disinterestedness, but upon the more solid foundations of science and social co-operation.

FAMILY BREAKDOWN

The case of the D. family illustrates the havoc caused by a too close relationship between mother and son. This case not only shows the vicious influence of in-laws and spiritualism but also the curative power of music and love.

In the grand strategy of nature the family has but one purpose: the nurture and preparation of the young for an independent life outside the family. Human beings differ from all other living organisms in one respect: our young infants are more helpless than the young of any other species, and they stay helpless for a relatively greater portion of their lives than the young of any other species. This means that the family, which is a temporary institution among other mammals, becomes a semi-permanent or permanent institution in human society. The farther we progress in the machine age, the longer it takes a human child to become mature and independent.

Incest, or the mating of members of a consanguineous family, is almost unknown among animals, because the temporary nature of the animal family and the early dispersion of its members makes incestuous attachments practically non-existent. In the human family, with its close and continued contact, incestuous relations are more likely to occur. Incest, however, is contrary to the law of nature, as it leads to the production of undesirable extremes, rather than the maintenance of a high general level of evolution. The result of inbreeding may be seen in domesticated dogs, where such diverse existing forms as huge Great Danes and tiny Mexican Chihuahuas can be traced to a common wolf-like ancestor. Such extreme types can result only from artificial inbreeding, as they do not occur naturally when animals live in the wild state.

The dangers of incest and its resultant effects of physical deterioration of the human stock are limited by social laws in all human communities, whether savage or civilised. But the dangers of the psychological equivalents of incest, the so-called psychological "fixations" due to the prolongation and intensification of family life have been recognised only in the last few years. It is almost inevitable that, when the family becomes a *goal* of life, as so frequently happens among socially isolated groups, rather than a *means* to the end of preparing the young for independent existence, the psychological preparation of the young for independent life will suffer in consequence. In our civilisation young men and women all too frequently find themselves incapable of normal adjustment to members of the opposite sex because they have, in the prolonged experiences of family life, established either complete satisfaction or rigid animosities in their relationship to their parents or siblings.[1] These abnormal attachments are usually due to the fact that the parents of the affected child have failed in their biological function as parents. By pampering, coddling, over-protection and over-solicitude, or by neglect, hate, arbitrary authoritarianism, they develop children who look at every man and woman outside the family either as an inferior or as a potential enemy.

These children, as they grow up, construct their sense of " face " entirely upon the approval of their families, or upon the love of some single member of their families. This attachment, as we have seen, may be of two types: either an abnormal attachment, amounting at times almost to sexual love; or, a pointed and bitter resentment often approximating to a vivid hate. A child may construct his entire

[1] A sibling is either a full brother or sister, i.e. any child of the same parents.

symphony of life upon the persistent melody of love or hate for a parent or sibling. We call the hated or loved parent the " contact-person ". The death or removal of such a contact-person represents a common critical situation. The psychological " fixation " often works its havoc on both members of the relationship. The parent is just as likely to suffer a breakdown as the child when such a vicious intra-familial fixation exists. The following analysis of the vicissitudes of the D. family will show how dangerous these fixations are, and how commonly they give rise to a nervous breakdown in one or several members of the family.

The D. family consisted of the father, an engineer, the mother, and the only child, Alfred, who was a musician of some repute. In the background are a number of the mother's relatives who hover on the neurotic periphery, always prepared to offer bad psychological advice on all family problems. Mrs. D. was the favourite child of her large family which was composed, almost without exception, of accomplished neurotics. All the women on mother's side were of the hovering broody-hen type, and most of the men, who were pampered darlings, were failures in the outside world. Mrs. D. escaped from this unwholesome atmosphere to marry Alfred D. (senior), a man of sterling worth and great objectivity, but without much experience in the handling of neurotic relatives. His life was embittered by the interference of his wife's numerous relatives, to such an extent that he had changed his profession so that he could spend considerable periods of time away from his wife. Nevertheless, he preferred the presence of his wife's relatives to being alone with his wife and her hysteria. The result was that when he was compelled to be at home he found the house over-run with relatives giving him gratuitous advice. His one goal in life was to keep his son from becoming a neurotic like the men in his wife's family. Mrs. D. lavished an inordinate amount of love on her son from the day he was born. The child was cursed with great physical beauty and a great musical talent, both of which were exploited *ad nauseam* by his mother and her relatives. The child scarcely ever had a moment of peace. He was constantly being admired and made much of and shown off before relatives and friends. He became such an impossible little prig that his father almost resented his presence as much as his precocity.

The father, recognising the fallacy of his wife's education of the boy, attempted to be strict with the child, and tried to compel him to play ball and "rough it". Water rolls down hill, and spoiled children sell their love to the highest bidder, gravitating toward the parent who pampers them most. Alfred (junior) developed a resentment toward his father, and preferred to bask in the adoring solicitude of his mother. The first nervous breakdown in the D. family occurred when Mr. D. insisted that Alfred should go to a boys' camp. Mrs. D. could not stand the thought that her darling child should be exposed to contact with rough and uncouth lads for an entire summer.

The father was adamant. Alfred went to camp amid the tears of his maternal relatives. Mrs. D. had to be removed to hospital. She had what seemed a heart attack, but the greatest heart specialists could find no organic cause for her symptoms. When she saw that the lad had actually been transported to camp, her cardiac symptoms vanished as if by magic. But she began to worry. She worried so professionally and so constantly that her husband finally had to capitulate and allow her to visit the boy at camp. The youngster had been making a fair adjustment under the expert guidance of those who were running the camp. As soon as his mother appeared on the scene there was an emotional drama without precedent in the history of the camp. All the good effect was nullified. Mrs. D. so completely disrupted the organisation of the camp that the child was sent home with her, after a week of anarchy, hysteria, and interference had affected the morale of all the other children and the staff.

The second breakdown occurred when young Alfred was sent to the university. This time again his father was adamant. The boy was to go to a " he-man's " college. Mrs. D. made a long journey to select her son's room, buy his furniture, rent his piano, establish his credit in the local shops. When her son went to the university she accompanied him, and kept him virtually a prisoner in her room at the hotel for a period of two weeks, lest he should be lost in his new surroundings. When she finally left him she had attempted to buy the affections of half the freshmen. Naturally, the boy was immediately disliked because he was a " sissy ", and was tortured more than his fair share by his fellow undergraduates, who not only agreed with his father's idea of " making a man of him ", but also shared the father's bad technique of accomplishing that end. After a month of agony, Alfred D. was back at home again. His father insisted that he should return to the university and see the thing through. Mrs. D. had another nervous breakdown, but Junior went back in spite of her tears, protestations and cardiac symptoms.

At the end of his first year at the university Alfred's father died suddenly of angina pectoris. Mrs. D. went into deep mourning and funereal hysterics. Alfred was not allowed to return to the university. He embarked intensively on his musical career, taking courses at the various musical foundations, practising for hours at home, and never leaving his mother. Now that her husband was dead, the mother intensified her affection for her son. They were always together. Mrs. D. literally feasted on the comments of her neighbours who said, " What a lovely relation between a mother and son! They are always together! " Alfred now became the helpless pawn of his mother and her relatives. His head was completely turned by their adulation. He was a good pianist, but to his relatives he was the best pianist in the world. Great preparations were made for his first public performance. Just before this recital Alfred had a miniature breakdown. His fingers became cramped. "Pianist's cramp," the doctor said, and as a result of this effective neurotic gesture that fatal test of personality was projected into the indefinite future. Mrs. D., in the meantime, became even more solicitous about her son's health.

After Alfred had recovered from his pianist's cramp, which is just another name for neurosis, he met one of the young women teachers at the music school where he was a first class pupil. She was his teacher in harmony. Alfred found himself falling in love with this young woman who was some five years his senior. He began taking her to concerts instead of always taking his mother. Once they went together to hear the performance of a new operatic cycle. Mrs. D. suffered a heart attack during the entire week-end. With uncanny precision her heart attacks always coincided with Alfred's expeditions with his new-found friend. When Alfred composed a Ballade and dedicated it to Edith, Mrs. D. thought the time had come for dramatic action. Subtly but unerringly, she set out to undermine Edith's position in her son's esteem. When two weeks passed without Alfred's seeing Edith, she sighed with relief. Now she was certain of her son. He would never fail her.

One day Alfred came home and unexpectedly

announced to his mother that he was engaged to be married to Edith. Mrs. D. fainted. She had hysterics, and suffered the most severe heart attack she had ever had. The doctor prescribed complete rest and a trip to the South. Alfred, of course, gave up his music and accompanied her. She improved rapidly under the influence of the balmy climate and the warm affection and solicitude of her son. As she improved he found an excuse to return home to his work and his Edith. He did not mention this last point, but his mother understood only too well. She threatened to take her own life if he left her in this, her greatest hour of need. Alfred remained another week. Then came the news that he had been engaged for a concert. He had to leave. Mrs. D. upbraided him for holding his personal ambitions more important than her welfare. But Alfred left, feeling independent for the first time in his life.

Mrs. D. was disconsolate. She was in the midst of her menopause. She could not withstand the pressure of enemies within and enemies without. In the course of her constant visits to specialists, a gynæcologist had discovered a non-malignant tumour, and had advised operation. Mrs. D. agreed to the operation, feeling that in submitting to the surgeon's knife she was suffering the martyrdom of a deserted mother. She went to the hospital outwardly brave and calm, but psychologically she was committing suicide. She had already relinquished life before the operation—her son had deserted her.

She died of surgical shock on the operating table, although she was in the hands of the most expert surgeon and anæsthetist. She had simply given up. She did not want to live.

When Alfred heard of his mother's death, and received the news from the surgeon that the operation could not be held accountable for her quick demise, he immediately sensed the psychological implication of his mother's death.[1] She had died of a " broken heart " as she had often threatened to do. Alfred looked about him. His maternal relatives accused him only too plainly of his lack of filial devotion. Some even overtly suggested that his want of consideration was the immediate cause of his mother's death. Her whole family was so completely attuned to her hysterical way of living that no one ever questioned the surgeon's or the anæsthetist's competency, but all immediately accused the son of having caused her death.

Edith tried to console him, but she became suddenly hateful to him. He broke his engagement with her. He returned to his musical studies, but could not bring himself to play the piano. His mother had died on a Thursday. He vowed that to the end of his days he would keep Thursday as a day

[1] Examples of so-called telepathy and telekinesis are not uncommon in cases like this where two people have been identified psychologically in a close symbiotic relation. When two vital rhythms are so closely contrapuntal, it is really not surprising that they should come to similar conclusions, even though separated by space.

of penance. He dressed only in dead black. On Thursday nights he burned two black candles in his study, and refused to answer the telephone, or eat, or see anybody. He assumed complete responsibility for her untimely death, and, haunted by a staggering sense of personal guilt, prayed for death to bring him both relief and atonement.

Alfred lost weight, complained of a constant pain in his chest, in the region of his heart (a symptom of identification with his mother's frequent cardiac pains), and spent most of the day and night reading old letters from his mother. He often thought of suicide as a means of joining her and ending his miserable existence without her. A friend suggested that he go to a famous spiritualist medium and attempt to " get in contact " with the deceased one. This Alfred did, spending a huge sum of money to have this medium " materialise " his mother. After some twenty unsuccessful attempts during which the medium assured Alfred that his mother was trying to get in touch with him, but was " just beyond the threshold " (during which time the medium doubtless gathered information about the mother and her habits, while collecting heavy fees), Alfred succeeded in " establishing contact ". By this time he was so hysterical that he would have been fair prey for the most arrant hocus-pocus. Once the " contact " was established, he lived only for the nightly conferences with the spirit of his dead mother. Dust gathered on the keyboard of his piano.

The medium finally spoiled her own game by letting the spirit of his mother voice the cryptic oracle, " Seek out thy first love and cleave to her! " Alfred interpreted this as advice to look up his former teacher and fiancée, Edith. Fortunately, Edith was an intelligent person with some psychological insight. She played her rôle cleverly, telling the young man that his mother had appeared to her in a dream and told her take her (the mother's) place in his life. Alfred still kept Thursday sacred to his mother's memory. He simply could not bring himself to do anything on that day. He worried all day Wednesday about what he would do on Thursday, and required most of Friday to recover from his melancholic sessions of remorseful introspection and self-castigation. Finally, Edith persuaded him to visit me in an effort to break the compulsion of keeping Thursday as a perennial day of mourning.

We must remember that Alfred had never had very much confidence in any man, especially in a man whom he could identify with the position of power and authority which he associated with his father. The first difficult task in this case was to establish a sympathetic relationship. This was gained by preliminary discussions of music and composition. I urged him to utilise the tragedy of his situation in the composition of a sonata tragica, thus linking his sorrow with an objective activity which would help to bring him out of his slough of despond. After the rapport was established, the next task was to remove him from the influence of his maternal relatives who still hovered about him like sad, long-faced pelicans. Alfred had enough insight by this time to agree to forbid his relatives all access to him. With the help of Edith he moved into a new studio, without giving his relatives his new address. The freedom from their psychopathic influence immediately helped his spirits to improve.

The Thursday mourning sessions continued until I suggested that a beautiful mourning cantata might be a more fitting monument to his mother than his isolation, black candles, and tears. To this, too, Alfred agreed, and the Thursday compulsion vanished as the cantata was begun. Little by little the psychological effect of his mother's solicitude was made clear to him, and as the history of his pathological family life unfolded, he began to see how his mother's solicitude was a form of tyranny, from which his father had died, and by means of which he himself had nearly been plunged into an unhappy life of neurotic grief.

Every effort was made to widen Alfred's social horizons. A young boy who had come to one of my clinics with a conduct problem had incidentally demonstrated great musical ability in the course of his treatments. He was designated as a special protégé for Alfred. For the first time in his life Alfred had someone to care for, instead of being himself the centre of all solicitude. The progress of this little pupil was one of the important new props to Alfred's growing self-esteem. Alfred began to practise and to compose with new vigour. He realised, himself, during the course of his psychological re-education, that he was free for the first time in his life.

As is often the case, the feeling of growth and psychic liberation became evident to him in a minor incident. One day he said to me, "You know, Doctor, I didn't realise how much I was tied to my mother's apron strings until this morning. I was leaving the studio, and suddenly ran back because I remembered that I had left some cigarette ashes in an ash tray, and mother always hated to have me smoke. She disliked even more having me leave cigarette ends and ash lying around the sitting-room when I left home. As I was running back to the apartment, I realised suddenly that I was free! My mother's pathetic look of disapproval would not greet me when I returned. I really did not have to go back. I could leave cigarette ends in the studio now without going through agony all day because of mother's disapproval. You cannot imagine how happy I was not to go back. You've made me a free man, Doctor!"

The story ends thus: the sonata tragica won a scholarship for Alfred, and, armed with fresh courage and insight, he has gone to Vienna for two years of study. And we can hope that the normalising influences of Continental life will finish the task of our psychotherapy. At any rate, Alfred's letters are full of a new joy in life. He gave his first concert in Prague without having a breakdown, and his latest compositions have won him great esteem. His road to mental health and happiness is clear.

MISCELLANEOUS BREAKDOWNS

After having read the case histories of the last three chapters, I hope the reader will have discovered that the nervous breakdown is not the mysterious disease it is supposed to be. The forms and symptoms vary from case to case, the critical situation is always different for each individual, and the physical constitution of the patient varies not only in each case but also in the same patient from day to day. But the laws of the nervous breakdown, as laid down in the first two chapters, hardly vary at all. In fact, we may say that all nervous breakdowns show a remarkable unity of structure, symptomatology, and purpose.

To be sure, we have not described the whole gamut of critical situations, and certainly not the whole gamut of symptomatology. Your own breakdown may seem unique to you, but the likelihood is that some psychiatrist has seen dozens of cases like it, and a careful and objective investigation will show that it follows the general scheme of all nervous breakdowns. Sometimes the breakdown occurs for apparently unaccountable reasons, and the treatment requires a tedious investigation of hidden psychological situations which are not apparent to the patient or to the family. In other cases everyone except the affected individual knows precisely what is the difficulty. The immediate cause of the breakdown may be some seemingly trivial failure which appears thoroughly innocuous to the onlooker, but is fraught with grave psychological consequences to the affected individual because of its deeper psychological implications to him.

Instances of this kind are not hard to find, and are very instructive. One young man had a nervous breakdown because, for the first time in his life, he received a " B " in an English course at the university. He had based his " face " on *exceptional* ability in English. He had lived a life of protest against his foreign-born parents who had never assimilated American culture. They still spoke with a marked Russian-Jewish accent. In his psychological pattern it was " up to him " to establish the famly honour by becoming an English professor at a university. The " B " was the first inkling that he could not be as completely successful as he had desired to be. The " B " which another student would have considered an excellent mark from this particular professor was tantamount to a failure to our patient.

Breakdowns are common in middle age. Usually some unimportant incidental physical ailment, the realisation that one cannot play golf as well as in former years, the appearance of a little paunch which some friend laughingly comments upon, the imputation that one is no longer " in such good form as usual ", or some similar trivial incident, may light the fuse that ends in a sense of complete hopelessness for the future. Often a remark of a child gives a parent the unmistakable feeling that he is *passé*, that he is no longer *au courant* with life, that he has become an " old fogey ". Vanities are touched, former abilities are waning, little fears of death creep in, and the critical situation is present. No major test or difficulty has appeared on the psychological horizon. The nervous breakdown is the first warning that the individual's " face " is threatened.

To some the critical situation comes in the form of leisure, enforced or earned. There are men and women who work all their lives to attain leisure, only to break down when they get it! One man had a nervous breakdown when he was compelled to retire from a company which he had formed, and for which he had fought all his life. On his sixty-fifth birthday he was presented with a scroll of appreciation, a fine gold watch and a release from his arduous duties as chairman of the company. The new chairman of the board did not realise that he had handed the " old man "—a critical situation: enforced leisure. Here was a man who had prepared himself for nothing but to fight all his life; a man whose " face " depended on winning a good battle. And now this laurel-wreathed veteran of countless economic battles stood inadequately armed before the one problem he could not solve: peace. Naturally, the cure consisted in putting him back into a fight; this time it was not just another economic battle, but a fight against juvenile delinquency. He began fighting for increased educational and recreational facilities for working-class children, for public playgrounds and community camps, for clubhouses and gymnasiums. In this manner he found his way back to health after three breakdowns. Anyone who understands the psychology of such a man could have predicted that rest, golf and travel, the first prescriptions that were given him, would not have the desired effect.

A common critical situation to occur is that of the man who has worked hard all his life but finds himself without economic security in old age. His children are grown up and independent. He is dismissed from his job because of his age. He is compelled to accept the charity of his sons and daughters, and to him this indicates failure, a loss of "face". His nervous breakdown serves as a justification: "I would not be dependent if I were not sick!"

Men and women who were famous on the stage or in the arts in their youth or maturity are often victims of nervous breakdown, when they must face the bitter reality that younger and more talented individuals have taken their places. We once treated a clown whose clowning no longer brought the laughs and plaudits of the crowd. He was dismissed from a travelling circus, a tragic and broken man. He regained " face " by teaching weaving and basketry to the blind.

Occasionally accidents or illness rob a man of the work for which he is best prepared, both psychologically and by training. The task of finding one's usefulness at a time when one's fingers are no longer nimble and one's reactions less plastic than in youth, often taxes the psychiatrist's resourcefulness, the patient's courage, the family's patience, or the social agency's funds. And yet in a world as full of occupations and activities as ours, some sphere of usefulness is open to everyone. Let those who see lead the blind; let the blind cheer the crippled; let the crippled console the poor; let the poor encourage the discouraged while they, in turn, can give solace or consolation to the blind. There is no situation so black or so hopeless that there is no help for it. There is no nervous breakdown so tragic that it cannot be cured. There is no inferiority feeling for which a useful compensation does not exist. There is no mistake so heinous that it cannot be at least partially rectified. There is no human being so badly off that he cannot find another in a worse plight if he seeks to find him. There is no critical situation which cannot be met, if not by conquest, at least by stoicism. A certain amount of stoicism is a valuable adjunct to human happiness. We often fall short of our ambitions, our plans go awry, our friends or loved ones disappoint us. Without a stoic disregard for these disappointments, life becomes a series of tragedies which no man can tolerate. The stoic " takes it on the chin ", and decides to keep on keeping on.

In the following chapter we shall examine the technique of cure. But before we proceed to our next task let us close this chapter with a motto, which that keen judge of human nature, Balzac, derived from an old Roman inscription in a physician's house—a motto which defines the task not only of the psychiatrist but of every human being. The motto is: *Guerir quelquefois, soulager souvent, consoler toujours*—to cure sometimes, often to relieve, and always to console.

CHAPTER SIX

PLAIN WORDS TO PATIENTS

Review of First Principles—A Decalogue for Patients —First Steps to Mental Health—The Cultivation of Awareness—The Cultivation of Social Responsibility —The Art of Empathy—The Technique of Social Life—Creative Self-Realisation

REVIEW OF FIRST PRINCIPLES

LET us assume that you have a nervous breakdown. The world looks very black to you, and you are tortured by intolerable symptoms. You have picked up this little book in the hope that in it you will find some magical cure for your troubles. Perhaps you have opened it at this very chapter because you are not interested in other people's cases and are impatient to get at the cure of your own condition. You are now eager for the curing word, the newest magical formula. You are hopeful and sceptical at the same time. You have been to dozens of " specialists " and have been disappointed in dozens of treatments. You have tried everything and you are still sick and discouraged. Cheer up. I have something very important to tell you.

Let us have a very personal chat, just as if you had come to consult me. Take me into a quiet place where no one will watch us or overhear our conversation. Sit down in the most comfortable chair you can find. If you smoke, take your favourite pipe, and light up. I'd ask you to do so if you were in my consulting room. If you like music, choose your favourite gramophone records and play them softly while you are talking to me, or turn on the wireless and get a good orchestra. Perhaps you prefer complete quiet. Relax. Take a few deep breaths. This will enable you to understand better what I am going to say. There! Now let's begin our talk.

If you are at all like the hundreds of other people who have come to tell me about their troubles in the past, you are looking for some magic cure for your difficulties. Perhaps you have tried a "faith" cure, auto-suggestion, hypnosis, or Christian Science, and have emerged from the experience more depressed and more bewildered than before. Perhaps you believe that psycho-analysis, by uncovering some unpleasant and forgotten event, will magically lift the mental fog in which you are groping for a way out. It's natural that you feel like this. People have sought for magic formulas since human beings began to think and to experience life. The will-to-believe is one of the strongest human impulses. The will-to-be-fooled is even stronger than the will-to-believe. You've been desperate. You must have help immediately. You are hoping against hope that you will find the magic formula for happiness in this book.

I want to be absolutely frank with you. I am no magician, no wizard, no miracle worker. I have no magic formula, and I cannot guarantee that you will be completely cured if you follow my advice. Any man who guarantees that he can " cure " a nervous breakdown is either an ignoramus, a deluded egoist, or a downright charlatan. I am only a doctor who has devoted his life to the healing of the mentally ill and the spiritually discouraged. In my experience I have discovered some truths and some techniques that have proved valuable in the treatment of cases like yours. These discoveries are not original with me. Some of them were known in ancient Egyptian medicine, and some of them go back even farther to the most primitive healing arts known to man. Hippocrates, the father of Greek medicine, wrote some of these things down long before the birth of Christ, and Moses Maimonides understood them and wrote wisely about them as far back as the twelfth century. Some of these truths have just been discovered in the last ten years, while others are as old as man. There is nothing magical about my advice. What I have to offer you is just common sense, the strongest, the soundest, the most magical of all healing forces.

Perhaps you are a little disappointed that I have no new and potent magic. Common sense seems such a dull way to approach a dramatic matter like a nervous breakdown. But do not be disappointed. Although I cannot guarantee to cure you, and still maintain my integrity as a physician, I can tell you this: if you follow the advice in these pages, there is every likelihood that you will *improve* your condition. The cure of a nervous breakdown is like the solution of a research problem by two scientists. One has all the facts at his command. The other has a technical procedure without which the facts cannot be mobilised or made useful to anyone. The man with the facts is discouraged because his facts have got out of control. He needs the technician badly. The technician knows he can help him. But the result really depends upon the speed with which the discouraged man with the facts puts these facts at the disposal of the technician. The more you collaborate and co-operate with me, the sooner your condition will improve.

The fact that you have read thus far in the book shows that you are willing to listen and to co-operate. It shows, moreover, that you have both enough insight to understand that something is wrong, and enough common sense to seek help. Thousands of people are walking the streets at this minute suffering from a nervous breakdown, too ignorant to know that something is wrong, or too stubborn or too proud to collaborate with an expert in affecting an amelioration of their condition. You belong to an enlightened fraction of humanity. This fact alone indicates that the chances are more than fifty per cent in favour of your getting well, even if you read no farther. The more you carry out the following suggestions, the quicker your condition will improve, and the happier you will be. That's encouraging, isn't it? There's no gain in deluding you with promises of a magical cure, and then letting you down, is there? Let us get to our job.

I want to review the salient points of my book with you for a moment. Let us define our troubles and our problems so that we will be speaking the same language. We have a few basic facts at our disposal. The first is that a nervous breakdown is not an accident, but an unconscious strategy of life, with a definite beginning in an inferiority complex; a definite, if unconscious, goal, i.e. the production of a feeling of security; and a well-defined technique, conscious and unconscious both, of attaining its goal. You remember that Nature watches over each one of us, and when she finds us going off the highroad of mental and physical health, she flashes her danger signals. These danger signals often take the form of physical symptoms referring to some specific part of the body. The greater the danger, the more insistent these danger signals are. The fact that you have symptoms, therefore, is a most valuable indication. It shows that you are reacting normally to a dangerous situation. No matter how intense or how unpleasant your symptoms are they must, therefore, be favourable signs of a curable condition. And that's another encouraging fact to work on, isn't it?

You will remember, also, that we are constantly looking at ourselves and comparing ourselves with other people for the purpose of building up a sense of "face". "Face" means simply our personal idea of self-esteem. We set up certain conditions under which we consider ourselves safe and secure in the eyes of our fellows. The maintenance of " face " is the basic profession of every human being. Life without " face " is intolerable. Some men and women, unfortunately and mistakenly, base their sense of " face " on untenable conditions. They want to be pre-eminent, first, impeccable, beloved by all the world, always in the centre of the stage, impregnably safe, perennially beautiful, or the like. No one can attain these false goals. The less valid we really think ourselves, the more of an impression we want to make. But you can see now that these high ideals are nothing more than the unconscious compensations for an unresolved inferiority complex. You find yourself in trouble sooner or later if you build up your sense of " face " on an impossible set of conditions. Nature warns you that you cannot pass the test. Reality threatens to tear the mask from your face. And presto! you have to have a nervous breakdown to " save your face "!

There are certain situations in life in which it is practically impossible to maintain a sense of " face " based on a false technique. We call them critical situations. Just before, during, or just after, such a critical situation has occurred, a nervous breakdown is most likely to happen. Just how the technique of the nervous breakdown is designed to maintain " face " was described in detail in Chapter II. The nervous breakdown sometimes effectually projects the critical situation into the indefinite future. Sometimes it accomplishes its end by the magical substitution of an "I cannot" for "I am afraid", and thus establishes an exoneration for your failure. The reason that you are unaware of what is happening in your nervous breakdown is that you cannot keep your "face", and know that you are evading the solution of a problem which everyone else must solve. The malingerer knows that he is afraid, and "fakes" a sickness. The nervous breakdown is a real sickness, whose mechanics are securely hidden in the depths of the unconscious. To deceive others, you must first completely deceive yourself.

I would never try to help you cure your nervous breakdown if it were not for one important fact: the nervous breakdown does not work! The nervous breakdown is a strategy of life which you have developed artistically and unconsciously. It is exquisitely appropriate to the unique task of maintaining your sense of "face" and it is uniquely suited to your individual constitution, your unique experiences of inferiority, your equally unique goal of security and superiority, and to the immediate critical situation which threatens you with a loss of your self-esteem. You are unaware of its mechanics, you are unconscious of its hidden goal, and you are ignorant of its origins. I may have given you a clue to its understanding, but before you read this book you were probably completely unconscious of what was going on in your life. Until you read the cases

I have cited you were probably completely unaware of the existence of painful experiences similar to your own. All you knew about your nervous breakdown was that, for you, it was a singularly painful and unpleasant experience, and that you knew exceedingly well. In fact you could hardly imagine that any doctor had heard of a similar case or that another human being had suffered agonies comparable to yours.

I do not know whether your nervous breakdown has really helped you to save your " face ". I do know that it is an ineffectual and terribly costly way of accomplishing your purpose. Originally the nervous breakdown is an unconscious mechanism, unconsciously chosen, and unconsciously operated for the purpose of " saving one's face ". But secondarily, it soon becomes a tyrant instead of a slave, a goal instead of a means. Sometimes it commits you to a life of invalidism, long after the original critical situation has passed. The unconscious, in its effort to effect its purpose, usually overdoes the nervous breakdown, just as nature, when she fills in a defect, over-compensates for the deficiency. To sum up: you unconsciously developed a nervous breakdown to rid yourself of an unpleasant responsibility, or to avoid a test of your personality which you feared would result in a loss of " face ". Viewed from this angle, your nervous breakdown was a form of social irresponsibility, a strategy of evasion.

But to-day you find that you are yoked to the

responsibility of keeping up your nervous breakdown. Your slave has become the most implacable of masters. You began by having a nervous breakdown. Now the nervous breakdown has you! Your responsibilities to the breakdown are worse than your responsibilities to nature and your fellow men. You alone can realise what the upkeep of a nervous breakdown costs. That is the reason I want to help you to cure yourself of it. Let us find out how we can give up the nervous breakdown, and work out a technique of maintaining your " face " more efficiently than by means of the painful symptoms of a breakdown. You have tried out an unconscious technique now for a long time. It has not brought you any happiness. Let us try a better method, a common-sense method, that has proved its value many times in the past. You have nothing to lose!

These facts about the nervous breakdown, which we have reviewed, enable us to face our mutual research problem of establishing your sense of " face " on a more reasonable foundation. They furnish us with a much more courageous outlook than if we were condemned to " muddle through " our task blindly. But I want to give you something definite to work upon, and here is a decalogue of conduct which you must learn to practise until it becomes quite automatic. You may not believe all the statements that I make, but that does not alter their relative truth. You have only your own experience and your " private logic " to fall back on, whereas these laws are the result of contact and experience with hundreds of nervous breakdown patients. I hope you are going to co-operate with me in this, and act " as if " these ten laws could guide you to happiness. Try them.

A DECALOGUE FOR PATIENTS

1. I have a nervous breakdown. This means that I have been swimming against the current of life, not with it. Nature has warned me (by giving me a whole galaxy of symptoms), that I cannot succeed in putting into practice my private ideas about the universe. I am going to take Nature's warning. It is unreasonable to believe that I can personally upset the laws of Nature. Fifty billion years of evolution can't be wrong.

2. The fact that I realise my plight is more than half the battle won. Instead of fighting against my symptoms, Nature's warning of danger, I am going to look for a better way of living. When I find this better way of living, the symptoms will disappear of themselves. Fighting against symptoms is a waste of time and energy. The first thing I am going to do about my symptoms is to stop talking about them to anyone. I shall try not to think about them, but if they do crop up from time to time I am not going to believe that I am having a relapse. A return of the symptoms is just a friendly warning from Nature to keep on keeping on.

3. My nervous breakdown is the result of my unconscious attempt to save my " face " by establishing a painful alibi for my personal failure. I am unaware of my own unconscious strategy because I have had to deceive myself before deceiving others. Now I have become a slave to my strategy of evasion. It demands greater and more painful responsibilities of me than I had bargained for. My nervous breakdown has only apparently effected its purpose. I am the loser by keeping it. Knowledge of my unconscious mechanisms is vital to my progress. My mis-education in the past is responsible for my present difficulties, but my knowledge in the present opens the way to new development in the future. What I do to-day will determine my future happiness. I am going to cease worrying about the past, and stop being afraid of the future. My problem is to live fully in the present.

4. Although I have perceived that my pattern of life was inadequate in the past, I have honestly not felt that I could make any change. My feelings are the result of my own unconscious attitudes. They are the result of my fears, my dreams, my mistaken ideas about myself and my past. My unpleasant feelings and fears were originally nature's warning signals. I have " lied with the truth " by unconsciously constructing them into arguments for not going on. I now know that I myself am responsible for these feelings, and I shall now act *as if* feelings were not arguments. No matter what my feel-

ings are, I am going to do what is right, what logic and science tell me are common sense. I have always said, " When I feel well I am going to do the right thing." This is putting the cart before the horse. I am now going to *do* the right thing, the common-sense thing first. This is an indispensable investment in happiness. When I have made my investment I will feel right, I will be happy.

5. My nervous breakdown is not an accident but the inevitable product of a muddled strategy of life. Even if it were an accident, it could not be cured by magic. It is ridiculous to believe that injections, gland treatments, rest cures, sedative pills, or sleeping potions can cure me. Neither can hypnosis, auto-suggestion, Christian Science, baths, massage, travel, " change of air ", or diet help me to overcome my difficulties. These are only the modern equivalents of the savages' magic incantations and rites. My nervous breakdown is really due to ignorance of the basic facts of life. It can be cured only by knowledge of what those facts are and by subsequent training along biologically normal channels. There is nothing wrong with my body, and nothing wrong with my mind. My difficulty lies only with my false ideals in life, my bad technique in living. I am going to try to be a better general of my vital forces. Others have succeeded. I also can succeed.

6. One of my chief difficulties has been the fact that I have been an extremist. My motto has always been "100 per cent . . . or nothing! " I have tried

to be God, and have failed. My critical situation made me fear that I would not realise my fantastic ambitions. In order to save my "face" I turned about and unconsciously tried to make a worm out of myself. The reason I have been unconsciously training to be an insignificant worm is that I have believed that no one could expect any social responsibilities of a worm. I am neither God nor an insignificant worm. I am a human being. Being an extremist is characteristic of infancy. In a grown-up world everything is approximate. No one is wholly white, and no one is wholly black. We are all shades of grey. I must make efforts to grow up. One way to grow up is to curb my personal ambition for power and security. Another important way of growing up lies in training my courage. The child is egoistic. The man is sure enough of himself to share his power with others. Strength grows from the conquest of obstacles. Failures are inevitable. No growth is possible without risking minor defeats. Running away from tests of my ability, however, leads to inevitable paralysis of my existing faculties. I will take a chance!

7. My nervous breakdown did not begin yesterday. It is the product of years of unconscious training. The reason that I did not break down before this is that I did not meet any critical test of my personality. I am glad that it came now, instead of later. It is inevitable that my progress towards normality will not proceed without difficulties. I will

not lose heart at minor setbacks. Relapses are minor incidents in growth. I am going to try to stop complaining about my hard lot, and I am going to try especially hard to refrain from beginning every statement with my old neurotic theme-signatures " if " and " but ". From now on my life is not going to be based on the formula " either . . . or " but on the new normalising formula " both . . . and! " No more alibis! I know I cannot undo the mischief of years of false living in a day. But there are years and years of happiness ahead of me if I change now. I will be patient and persevering.

8. During my nervous breakdown I have been seeking a scapegoat to blame for my failures. I, as a person, am now responsible for my future success. There may have been factors in the past that can explain my deviations from the normal. Everyone has discouraging experiences. Everyone misses some of his opportunities. Everyone is sometimes frustrated by the innate perversity of inanimate objects. But all these discouragements, while they can explain my present, cannot compel me to remain in this condition, either in the present or in the future.

9. All during my nervous breakdown I have been working in the fog of the unconscious. I did not realise the sources of my inferiority feeling because I was too young to understand them when they were formed. I did not realise my unconscious goal of superiority and security because these things were never taught me at school. I did not conceive that I

have really been spending my life in an unconscious profession: keeping up my "face". I still want to keep my "face", because life without self-esteem would be intolerable. But now I understand that the only real security and the only real satisfaction of life consists in an ideal of "face" based on service to my fellow men. To this end I must develop my personality to the widest limits that I am capable of attaining. From to-day on I am going to approach this problem in the light of my conscious understanding, instead of muddling through by the uncertain glimmer of unconscious motivations. My human ability to mobilise my conscious forces is what distinguishes me from a worm or a cow. The good life consists in utilising the tremendous energy of the unconscious for the attainment of conscious, rational, and socially useful goals.

10. This is the end of my nervous breakdown. So long as I was ignorant of true facts and right values, I was really not responsible for my pattern of life. Now I know what the facts are. No matter how long I have been running up the wrong street, I have lost nothing but a little time. In fact my unhappiness will make me appreciate the joys of complete living all the more. I know the truth, and the truth has made me free. From this moment I am going to be the captain of my own soul, the master of my destiny. My happiness will be the sweeter for knowing that I have attained it on my own responsibility. It is easier to be normal than to be neurotic. From this

day on I am going to take the material that Nature has given me and hew it into a beautiful design. I have always been asking of Life, " What do I get out of it? " From now on I am going to become an artist in the fine art of living completely. My question now is, " What can I put into it? " As part of my new programme of living I am going to increase my awareness of the world about me. My nervous breakdown has been due to a restriction of my horizons. I have been dying of spiritual suffocation. I have built a vault about myself to keep out dangers, and I have only succeeded in keeping out the sun, the good fresh air, and the smiles and encouragement of my fellow men. All that is human is my province. I have been doing nothing but complaining of my miserable feelings, and torturing myself with doubts and fears. From this moment I am going to seek my salvation in outside activities. Nothing has come of my breakdown but pain and more symptoms. From now on I am going to direct my energies to living a life of freedom, of reason, of expression, and of altruism. Nothing could be worse than my breakdown. I have nothing to lose, everything to gain.

Now you have your decalogue. I want you to read it over every day, morning and night, until you can almost recite it. You say you are not interested in developing yourself or in devoting yourself to altruistic tasks? You want relief from your symptoms. If I could wipe the slate of your past clean, free you immediately from your symptoms, and put you in an entirely new environment where no one would know you or your past, believe me, I would do it. But you yourself know that this is impossible. You must make this first step alone. I am here to guide you, to help you, to encourage your efforts, to cheer your success. Did you ever get dividends from a bank without first making a deposit? No! And you cannot get relief from your symptoms without making an investment in living. Take a deep breath, and we'll begin!

FIRST STEPS TO MENTAL HEALTH

The first thing you must do is to put a little order into your life. Make out a schedule for to-morrow. Begin with a brisk walk, or exercises if you like them. Sit down to breakfast and read your morning paper over a cup of good coffee. You've been neglecting your appearance lately. Get your hair cut, have your nails manicured, a face massage, or a permanent wave to-day. Put on a new tie, a new dress, new gloves, a new hat, your best clothes. If you haven't bought any new clothes recently, put that on your programme. You'll feel better if you're in the fashion—so long as the fashion is reasonable. Get the latest issue of some first-class weekly, and find out what your neighbours in the world have been doing while you have been complaining about your symptoms. See whether you cannot get interested in some human problem that is raised in their pages. Try to smile at the lift man. If anyone asks you how you feel, answer, " Much better, thank you! " and say it with a smile. Do not discuss your symptoms with anyone.

If you have a business, go down and look the office over. Get a humorous magazine on the way and learn a funny story. Tell that story until you make someone laugh. That's your first job. Then have lunch with an old friend whom you've been neglecting. Don't broadcast your troubles. Ask him about *his* life, and see whether you can cheer him up. Give him some good advice, make him laugh. Convince this man that you are coming out of your recent illness, and have a new zest for life.

Of course I know that you cannot do all of these things. You may be living on a lonely farm, or you may be a typist with just a shilling for lunch. Get the spirit of my advice—not the letter. You must use your imagination, and adapt my counsel to your own needs. I am not a clairvoyant. I cannot foresee the specific situation in which you find yourself. I wish we could talk it over face to face. But since I am not actually sitting beside you, I know you will take my advice in the spirit in which it is given. I am really trying to make just one point. You will never get well sitting at home, stewing in your own juice. You won't find any cure for your breakdown by vigils of introspection or long hours of broadcasting your symptoms. Get out and do something, see something, feel something of the world going on about you. An ivory tower is a lovely place to have a nervous breakdown. It is no place to get well. Come out of your ivory tower!

This afternoon go to a cinema, a matinée, a concert, or an art gallery if there is one you can visit. If you live in the country, get out for a long walk. Be certain that you accost someone and start a conversation. It doesn't really matter whether you ask your neighbour the time, or the way back to your own house. I want you to listen to human voices. You've been a hermit much too long. Perhaps you can tell your funny story to someone. Keep on the look-out for someone you can help. A smile, a hearty handshake, a word of encouragement are all you need to start.

In the evening, if you cannot join some group of people, sit down with a good book or listen to the wireless. Telephone a friend you have not seen for some time, and make a date. Ask him how his dog or sick aunt is getting along. If you have nothing better to do, read over any parts of this little book which may not have been quite clear to you on first reading. If you like, you can sit down and write me your life story, and thus hold an intimate conversation with me. You can always do that if you are lonely. Then go out for another walk before going to bed. Try to repeat as much of my decalogue to yourself as you can. And put yourself to sleep thinking about it, planning to put it into execution.

So much for your first day. From now on I want you to attempt to expand your horizons a little every day. After your first few days I want you to make it a rule to do two things. First, seek the opportunity to be helpful to someone every day. Second, seek the opportunity to do one thing you've always been afraid of doing every day. It does not matter how you are helpful, or what fear you overcome. The purpose of being helpful to others is to give your own individuality a chance to expand. The purpose of conquering a fear a day is to demonstrate to yourself that 99 and 44/100ths of the things you have been afraid of never happen. If you cannot help someone, imagine how you would have helped someone if the opportunity had presented itself. Be prepared to help. If you cannot overcome a fear, rehearse your fear-laying conduct mentally, so that you will be ready when the opportunity comes.

The moment you start expanding your personality you are going to feel better. This will be gratifying to you. Perhaps it will be so gratifying that you will rest on your oars and cease working out your problem. Then the symptoms will return, and you will be discouraged and give up the good fight. Your worst suspicions will be confirmed. You will be certain that there is no real cure for *you*. I am warning you against such tricks on yourself. If you give up you are fooling no one but yourself. Remember, symptoms are not arguments. I do not expect you to accept everything I say or advise without making some mental reservations. I want you to be scientifically sceptical, but you have been on the wrong track for a long time. Your neurotic technique is well developed. It has attained a certain moment of inertia, to use an engineering term. I do not expect that you are going to change overnight, by magical metamorphosis, into a different human being. You are now in the period of transition. It may be that your symptoms *are* actually worse than they were when you first started reading this book. But that is no reason for not " keeping on ".

As a matter of fact, if your symptoms get worse after you attempt to carry out my advice, you may be certain that I have hit the bull's-eye. I have made the right diagnosis and touched your Achilles heel! Your unconscious will now start playing tricks with you. You will " lose " this book, mislay it, or actually throw it away. You will wish you had never heard of me. You will have worse symptoms and fears than ever before. If you were coming to consult me you would probably come late to your appointments, or refuse to pay me for my services, or punish me by having bad dreams about me. As it is you will probably say very mean things about this book to yourself, and make mental reservations about its veracity. All these signs of what we psychiatrists call resistance only signify that we have come to the heart of the problem. And it hurts. Your resistance is just another way of saving your " face " by avoiding the implications of my counsel.

You will again begin to hanker after magic cures. You will be too tired, or too disinterested, or too sick, to go on with my precepts. Our little conversation will have become just another critical situation for you. And you will try to run away and hide your head in the sands of the unconscious just like the poor maligned ostrich in the fable.

Now why run away from the truth? Running away will not alter the facts. The facts are inescapable. What I am suggesting to you, a normal life, is really the easier way. It's certainly much simpler than having a nervous breakdown. You cannot run away now because one piece of magic has already been accomplished. If you have read thus far I am afraid I have given you a bad conscience. I have disclosed your own unconscious mechanisms of flight or rage to you. You cannot now go back to your old unconscious technique, because a nervous breakdown can only "work" when you do not understand *how* it works. But now you already have some insight. You cannot go back, because if you do you will lose "face", you will know you are cheating. You may be afraid of going forward. But, really, you have nothing to fear. The good life is the easiest and most satisfying life. So cheer up, and let's go on!

I did not really want to frighten you with this description of resistance, but if you know about it in advance you will save yourself a great deal of useless discouragement. Now that we have made up our minds to go forward, we need a *conscious* plan. I want you to think about a Five-Year Plan for yourself. Not just a plan of getting more money, or more power, or more love. A plan that will be a combination of internal growth and development and of eternal expanding usefulness to mankind. You may be a practical, extroverted, " go-getting " individual whose breakdown was the result of overweening ambition, or you may be a quiet, contemplative, introverted soul, whose breakdown was the result of faint-heartedness. Naturally, I do not want to make a robot of you. The suggestions that I am going to make must of necessity be rather general. You must choose those suggestions which most closely fit your constitution, your training, your environment.

The suggestions I shall make may be applied at various levels of human activity. If you are a retail grocer with a secondary school education and I suggest that you expand your social horizons, by joining some local club or society, this may be just the thing that is going to bring you out of retirement. At the same time, if you are a Professor of Archæology at a great University, and I suggest that you come out of the cloistered seclusion of scholastic life, I shall expect you to do so by identifying yourself with the League for Industrial Democracy, the World Peace movement, or by lending your services for the establishment of exchange scholarships. The psychological benefits in each case will be quite comparable.

THE CULTIVATION OF AWARENESS

You have a nervous breakdown. That means that you have been following a path which could be described graphically by an "ingrowing spiral". You have been constricting your social, mental, sexual, occupational and recreational horizons little by little, until all that remains is your own body and your own thoughts. The human mind, operating in a normal way, in the solution of external problems, works smoothly and imperceptibly. The mind is a tool designed to help us attain our goals of security and self-realisation. Torn from its normal activities, the mind ceases to be a good tool, and becomes its own goal. Instead of thinking how you could better your vital situation, you have been thinking about nothing but your own thoughts. The process of thinking in itself is not a valid problem to anyone but a psychologist or philosopher. If your own thoughts are the goal of your thinking, and those thoughts are normal thoughts, they are extremely uninteresting. In order to keep yourself from being bored to death, therefore, you have had to make your isolated thought life interesting by developing all kinds of phobias, obsessions, delusions, illusions, or even hallucinations. You have been afraid of being afraid, anxious about your own anxiety, deluded by your own delusions. These mental processes, however "normal" and expected in a nervous breakdown, are not part of the process of getting well. Our first task, therefore, is to put those thoughts back where they belong, at the job of making life more interesting and enjoyable.

One of the first things that I advise you to do, therefore, is to cut some windows in the mental and spiritual vault in which you have locked yourself. Throughout your breakdown you have been defending yourself frantically against the imaginary enemy of reality. Reality is your friend, not your enemy. The more you know about reality the less interested you will be in having a nervous breakdown. Think of it! You are living in the most interesting, the most thrilling, the most intellectually exciting age that man has ever known. Science, art, economics, technology, politics and education are all in a ferment. New ideas, new techniques, new discoveries, new philosophic concepts are being born every day. The depression challenges our smug economic theories, technocracy throws the gage to politics, crime threatens to overwhelm our police systems, communism in Russia gives the lie to our hallowed beliefs in " rugged individualism ". Science questions our very concepts of matter and space, the Church totters, and psychology denounces the holiest beliefs of the law and education. The whole world is in the most cataclysmic turmoil. The daily newspaper chronicles events fully as thrilling as those of the Terror of the French Revolution. And in the midst of all this excitement, all you do is think about your headache, your palpitating heart, your depression, your timidity, your sorrows! Men fly from Coast to Coast, braving wind and weather, in less than a day, and you are afraid to ride in the subway! Einstein scrambles the stars, giving us a new cosmos, and you are preoccupied with a sense of guilt for acts that few know and no one will remember!

Open your eyes to what is going on about you! Take those lectures you have been wanting to attend for such a long time. Read a good book review column in one of the better newspapers or magazines, choose a book, buy it and read it. Get acquainted with your public library. The librarian will be only too glad to advise you on a course of reading. Learn a new language if you can. Sign up for some extension courses in one of the greater universities. If you live in or near a big city all kinds of institutions and foundations offer interesting and provocative intellectual fare to suit your special needs or predilections. A night school may have just the answer to your problem. Learn how to typewrite, learn how to drive a car, take dancing lessons, music lessons, language lessons, art lessons! It matters little which you choose. But do *something* to expand your horizons and put yourself in touch with the majestic throb of humanity.

Never before have the better magazines offered such stimulating articles. They will open a new world of contemporary thought to you. Choose one or two of them and read them assiduously as part of our programme of getting well. You say you cannot concentrate? This is a fallacy. Just think how hard you have been concentrating on your symptoms! You are a virtuoso in concentration. You must only *direct* your concentration to the outside world. You are bored with your own symptoms by this time. You concentrate so hard on the futile process of chasing your own thoughts and feelings around in a circle that your brain is tired. Half of this amazing mental energy of yours, if spent in learning about international politics, if occupied in investigating the wonders of science and invention, or in reading the good books, old and new, that you have neglected to read, will bring you incredible dividends in pleasure, relaxation and recreation.

Cultivate your awareness. Come out of your vault of defensive egoism and get into the most exciting drama the world has ever seen. Get into the great human parade. It is not nearly so difficult as being a slave to a nervous breakdown. What, you are not interested? This is another fallacy. You cannot get interested in the world without making an investment. A moron is not interested in archæology, because he lacks the mental equipment to be interested. But you have a nervous breakdown, and that's evidence that you possess sufficient mentality to be interested. But you cannot get interested in the world if you shut your eyes to what is going on. You must follow this advice, even if it hurts. Remember, feelings are not arguments. The more you know, the easier it will be to get well. The more you study, the sooner you will get off your " ingrowing spiral " and begin the process of personality expansion. Awareness is the beginning of creative self-realisation. Creative self-realisation is what I want to teach you.

The more you know, the more quickly you attain an objective realisation of your own value. All your life you have been comparing yourself with people. You've been afraid that some of them were far superior to you, while those who were inferior did not interest you. Stop comparing yourself with people, and begin finding out something about this interesting world you are living in. Begin living in it. Begin finding your place and your value in it. Expand your personality by cultivating your awareness. Without extensive awareness your sense of " face " cannot be secure.

THE CULTIVATION OF SOCIAL RESPONSIBILITY

All your life you have been playing the rôle of the lone wolf. In order to keep your ego safe from harm you have isolated yourself and built all kinds of walls about yourself. Society has made a great investment in you. Your fellow men kept you alive when you were sick. They educated you. They protected you from the depredations of socially irresponsible individuals. They cleaned your streets, purified your water, built your house. Thousands of generations of men have given you their supreme heritage, the written word, the published result of their daring discoveries. Men allowed themselves to be burned at the stake so that you might walk down the street and worship in any church or temple you choose. Men offered their lives so that you might ride in safety in the underground, turn on the electric light, or take your favourite headache powder, without harm to yourself.

The older the world becomes, the more the social interdependence of all human beings is established. Time was when millions could die of famine in China while you ate your breakfast bacon in complacency. To-day the wireless flashes the news of disaster to every corner of the earth within a few minutes of its occurrence. It immediately touches your problems. What with the constant psychological and sociological shrinkage of the world, every man's problem is every other man's problem. You cannot escape this fact. Perhaps the reason for your former isolation, your hankering after self-protection, your suspicion of your fellow men, can be found in your ignorance of the meaning of social relations, your bad training in the art of making friends, your exaggerated expectations of human virtue, or your emotional demands on people. Whatever the cause, you see now that isolation can lead only to unhappiness.

Unconsciously you have been going through life

with a chip on your shoulder. People have not treated you right. But in all probability you have not realised that people's attitudes toward you were the result of your own unconscious attitude toward them. Your misanthropic attitude expresses itself in your gait, your handshake, your facial expression, without your being in the least aware of its existence. And men are imitative creatures. If they read your unconscious misanthropy (whether expressed by hesitation, timidity, withholding, or by actual hate and dislike) from your unconscious attitudes, they will also quite unconsciously mirror their perceptions in their actions. They will treat you, unconsciously, as you expected (again unconsciously) to be treated. The result is that your worst fears have often been confirmed, and you have come to the final conclusion that men and women are not to be trusted. The result of this vicious circle is continued isolation, resentment, and deepened misanthropy. This kind of unconscious muddling is all very well if you want to retain your nervous breakdown, but if you want to be happy, you must now mobilise your *conscious* thinking and behaviour for the attainment of the new goal of creative self-realisation in service to your fellow men.

All virtue and achievement, all fame and self-realisation are by-products of man's social life. Every individual's sense of " face " depends, finally, upon social values, upon social approval. I do not mean by this that you must adapt yourself to all of the local or temporary insanities which characterize your family, social group, or national government. I mean that you must find your own sense of " face ", your own sense of value, by being true to the best in the human tradition. You cannot otherwise be true to yourself. If you have not succeeded in the technique of being all that a human being can be, do not be discouraged. We have learned how the stars move in their courses, how rivers can be harnessed to the needs of a lemon grove, how the lightning may be tamed and the air conquered by ponderous machines, but the science and art of being human are still in their infancy. Those who were responsible for your lack of education in this important sphere of learning, or even responsible for your active mis-education along these lines, were probably doing the best they knew how to do at the time. At any rate, there is no time to waste resenting your defects or in beating your breast mourning for lost time. You must begin now to learn how to be happy in being as nobly human as you can be.

The first thing to remember is that you are not alone in this leaking life-boat which we call civilisation. We are all going to sink or survive together. Your problems are also your neighbour's problems. You have always thought that your inferiority complex was the worst in the world, but I assure you that we all have our weak and tender spots. If you would only remove the blinkers from your eyes, you would see that there are a great many people in the world worse off than you are. And many of those who seem to have all the things that you want have other problems that are not visible on the surface. The street-cleaner envies the bank president, but the bank president envies the anonymity which is symbolised by the street-cleaner's uniform. The timid soul envies the loud assurance of the " go-getter ", but all the time the " go-getter " is in mortal terror lest someone discover that he is whistling in the dark.

THE ART OF EMPATHY

One of your first tasks, therefore, in the process of creative self-realisation which will lead to the cure of your breakdown, is to find the way to your fellow man. To this end you must cultivate all the arts and techniques that bind man to man. The first of these is the art of identification. Love, sympathy, fellowship, charity, social responsibility, social vision follow identification, or empathy, as we psychiatrists call it, as the night follows the day. The average human being, blundering through his social life, does not take the time to identify himself with his fellow men. It is much easier to dispose of them by attaching a convenient label. Thus we find people saying of others that they are not socially " right ", or that they lack " personality ", or that they are rascals, saints, fools, or sinners. To call anyone a name may be a convenience but it does not help human understanding. Wars are fought because this process of labelling men instead of understanding them turns into national politics. Fifty million Germans cannot all be bad, fifty million Frenchmen cannot all be wrong, fifty million Americans cannot all be right. Neither is a man who does charity necessarily a saint, nor a man who steals necessarily a born or a confirmed criminal.

If you want to understand people—and life is not worth living if you are continually in the wrong about people's motives, actions, beliefs or desires—you must identify yourself with them. This means that in approaching any human being you must do so with the premise that if you had the same sense of inferiority, the same education or mis-education, the same goal in life, you would be doing exactly as he is doing. When you have this feeling as a basis, you can deal correctly with anyone. Remember, every human being not only has a basic sense of inferiority, but every human being is trying to get rid of his sense of inferiority and establish his " face " and his security. You may not subscribe to his technique, but you can try to understand it.

Every teacher, prophet, comedian, doctor, general, prize-fighter, showman, salesman, or business executive who merits the name of *great* derives his greatness from his ability to understand human beings, from his desire to identify himself with their fundamental conduct, their vanities and their ambitions, their motives, goals, and their individual techniques. If you cannot identify yourself, you will constantly be in social hot water. If you have no empathy, you will always be talking about ropes in the hangman's house, about death in the home of the sick man, about divorce in the living-room of the unhappy wife. Social tact is another name for identification. But tact is only the passive side of identification. Empathy implies an active participation and an active encouragement of every human being you meet. And more. It implies the active seeking out of individuals who need your help and your encouragement.

The technique of identification is easy. Instead of looking at every man's most obvious defect, look for an asset and compliment him on it. Mr. John Smith is considered a lazy and irresponsible man. If you tell him this to his face, he will hate you, and unconsciously attempt to revenge himself on you for your assault on his sense of " face ". But Mr. Smith has a very nice tree in his front yard. You know he is inordinately proud of this tree. You say to him, " What a wonderful tree! You must have cared for it with a great deal of love to have it flower so beautifully. My uncle has a similar tree in his front yard but it does not bloom nearly as well. You must be an expert gardener! " What happens? Mr. Smith immediately makes a mental reservation that he is going to cultivate that tree. It gives him significance. His wife has been telling him for months to get out a spade and liven the roots. This implied his laziness, and he resisted to maintain his "face". But after your comment Mr. Smith not only decides to dig round his tree, but his opinion of you immediately goes up several points because you have had the good sense to appreciate his magnolia tree.

Noblesse oblige. Instead of maintaining his belief that you are a crabbed old codger who plays bad bridge, he becomes interested in you as a sympathetic personality. " How is your charming wife? " he asks you, and immediately you feel proud that someone shares your opinion of your wife. A better feeling has been engendered between you and Mr. Smith. With a little cultivation it may ripen into a friendship. Mr. Smith will recommend some of his customers to you as clients, and you will think of Mr. Smith when your client complains that his roof is leaking. Mr. Smith will do a fine job of roofing in order to corroborate your good opinion of him. Little by little Mr. Smith will consider you his good friend, and you find that Mr. Smith is not the idler he was supposed to be, but a very delightful dinner guest and golf companion. All by a small initial investment in the technique of identification.

Or, you believe that Mrs. Jones is a malicious gossip. She has carried tales about you to neighbours. You hate her and fear her sharp tongue. But you know that Mrs. Jones makes delicious raspberry preserves. You pack up your pride and your suspicions and pay Mrs. Jones a visit. Let her talk, but do not be too interested in her gossip. You know she gets a sense of power and bolsters her " face " by being the first to tell you that Mrs. Doe has a lover, and that Mrs. Goldstein's children use obscene language. Shift the subject to household matters. Let her know that her reputation as a raspberry preserver has spread into the far provinces. You beg her for her formula, her special technique. *Noblesse oblige.* Mrs. Jones will share her secrets with you. You assure her that there must be something else, something truly individual that makes her preserves so much better. Mrs. Jones glows and expands. She invites your Johnny to come and play with her Jack in his sandheap. She compliments you on the fine way you have brought up your children. She has become your friend, instead of your enemy. You haven't lost anything and you have extended your social horizons.

It makes no great difference what social or professional status you occupy. The same technique works with princes and paupers, with professors and plumbers. There is the example of a young colleague who once came to a capital city to practise in a very difficult medical special subject. There was only one outstanding man in that subject in that city. He was known in the profession as a "difficult" person. In due course word got around to my young friend that he was being libelled and defamed by this older man wherever the older man had an opportunity to do him damage. My young friend was advised by his lawyer to prefer charges against the older physician before the grievance committee of the Medical Association. My counsel was that he should identify himself with the older man's position. It was obvious that the younger man's brilliant work was a threat to the older man's sense of professional " face ". " You will probably outlive him," I told my colleague. " Why not have him for a friend instead of an enemy? I know it is not your fault that he has a mote in his eye, and I sympathize with your difficulties. But try my way. Make it your business to praise him on every possible occasion. Quote his works when you write, quote his words when you speak. His ego is now your worst enemy. Make it your best friend. Any man with such an inflated ego is vulnerable. Kindness will deflate him faster than harsh words." The young man followed my advice. Echoes of his praises came to the older man. From every side he heard nothing but reports of the younger man's good will toward him. *Noblesse oblige* for the noble. *Faiblesse oblige* for the inferior. The older man's further criticism was inhibited by his own vanity. Identification, you see, is not only a positive aid in the extension of social horizons. It is also an indispensable defence against the neurotic misanthropy of others, where such misanthropy unhappily exists. In either case, the practice of empathy can lead only to beneficial results.

Did I hear you mumble an objection? Something about insincerity, something about your refusal to tell such lies, to flatter people when they do not deserve it? My friend, sincerity and truth are very relative terms. The child, the savage, and the neurotic follow a philosophy of opposites. For them right is right, and wrong is wrong. To the adult, all things are relative and approximate. If there is any absolute truth, then that truth is the fact that human beings cannot live without one another. Anything, therefore, that improves human relations must be true and good. Better a little insincerity among friends than the unadulterated truth between enemies. No one can really bear the absolute truth. That's why we all carry masks before our faces, that's why we camouflage our conduct, that's why we work so hard to maintain our " face ". Any little insincerities that occur in the course of your carrying out my suggestions are really closer to the truth than your usual unpleasant blurting out of unpleasant facts. No matter. Take this as a piece of friendly and practical advice. It is better to be insincere and friendly in little things, while maintaining rigid honesty in the things that count, than to be absolutely honest in little things, and live a life whose entirety is a lie. If you must be absolutely honest, apply your ideas to scientific research or politics where absolute honesty is an asset. In your human relations temper your sincerity with the milk of human kindness. Human beings are frail and imperfect vessels. Encourage them, and judge them not too harshly.

THE TECHNIQUE OF SOCIAL LIFE

After you understand the philosophic and psychological meaning of empathy, go out and practise it. Every man, woman and child has a story. You used to ride in a tubeway or bus and feel that everyone was looking at you with hostile eyes. Now begin to look at those fellow passengers with your new technique. Try to imagine what their background is, what their goal of life. Spend your time asking yourself to what end you would logically act if you were acting as they acted. You will see how quickly your symptoms disappear, and how quickly the time flies.

And now I am going to give you a task. Make a chart of the days of the week, and divide the space for each day into two parts by drawing a vertical line through the middle. On the left of each day's compartment you will make a mark for every good deed, every encouraging word, every good story you have told, every time you have identified yourself with someone and tried at least to make him a little happier. On the other side of the dividing line in each day's space, you will place a little cross mark for every unfriendly act and every omission or inhibition of human interest. I am not really interested in the cross marks. I want them to be a stimulus to you because this prescription I have just given you is the first step in creative self-realisation. And if you have no opportunity to do your good deed, put that down as a cross. It means you have not looked hard enough. I do not care whether you only slap the lift boy on the back, whether you tell your maid a funny story, whether you bring your wife some flowers, or whether you actually give away your overcoat to a poor man. The least you can do is to take down your telephone and call a friend you have neglected, or buy an unemployed man a cup of coffee. And by the way, thinking how you are going to carry out my prescription is the best sleeping medicine in the world. Don't count sheep. Try to recount ways of being human.

A good way to begin your practise of social empathy is to begin with individuals who are already submerged by our machine civilisation. Children, old men and women, "wall-flowers", the unemployed, lift boys, postmen, domestic servants, bus conductors, and the like, should be the objects of your first experiments. Every man has a story. Every human being is a potential broadcasting station. All you need to do to get a man's story is to make it obvious that you are sympathetic or "tuned in". The most valuable single asset in the art of being a good human being is the ability to listen intelligently and sympathetically. Unfortunately, you have been so preoccupied broadcasting your own woes that you haven't had time to listen to anyone else. But from now on you must listen, and learn.

Oh, yes, I know your objections, because I take

my own medicine and have identified myself very keenly with you in your present situation. You are saying, " Dr. Wolfe, how can you expect me to make other people happy when I'm so unhappy myself? " The same old egoism and self-centredness, isn't it? You are putting the cart before the horse. Make other people happy to the limit of your ability, and your own happiness will accrue in the course of your activity. Now may I ask you a question? How can you expect to be happy when you spend all your time broadcasting your troubles? You must begin by being something of a Stoic, and make this mental reservation: No matter how I feel, I will listen to someone else's trouble. And if I listen long enough, I may find some way to help him out. In this way I can find a valid goal for my own life, and thus find a sense of self-realisation in helping another pilgrim on this hard road.

After you have tried your technique of empathy on your relatives, friends, servants, you must begin to form some acquaintances with strangers. I mean, talk to the people sitting next to you at a concert, talk to the strangers viewing pictures at an exhibition, waiting with you in a queue at the theatre, or riding beside you in a bus or a tube. The likelihood is that these people will have somewhat similar goals, and will entertain your questions cordially. I can hear the sticklers for propriety bristling at such a suggestion. " That sort of thing isn't done! " they say scornfully. Very well. Our prevailing social traditions are stultifying. They are responsible for the fact that we look at the average stranger as we would at an alien enemy. To what good end? If you follow the prevailing codes, the best that you can do is to develop some form of social and intellectual snobbery. This type of snobbery is responsible for the propagation of more and more neuroses, more and more nervous breakdowns! Do not be afraid. If someone rebuffs you, you can put him d wn as a worse neurotic than you are. The greatest human beings are always the most modest, the most kindly, the most willing listeners. This applies equally to men and to women. The social conventions which forbid speaking with a fellow human being were written by neurotics as measures of self-defence.

The technique of making the acquaintance of strangers is generally abetted by the existence of certain common subjects of conversation such as the weather, politics, sport, the health of relatives, and the state of business. Do not scorn these subjects of conversation, which, although they may themselves be unimportant, pave the way to more intimate subjects. Many a lasting friendship has grown up out of casual conversations about the weather. If you can afford to do so, go on a sea voyage. Steamship travel is an admirable opportunity for the creation of new interests and friendships. The peculiarly favourable psychology of a ship lies in the fact that most people forget their prejudices and their social defences when they get beyond the three-mile limit. On board ship humanity becomes crystallised. The intimate social life that develops at sea, together with the passengers' physical isolation from their usual bases of supply (and prejudice) are well calculated to teach men and women how much they depend upon their fellow men. Sharing your morning soup with your neighbour in the next deck chair, or dancing with an utter stranger, or eating with a native of another country three times a day, usually breaks down one's tendencies toward clannishness and insularity, and opens the way to the establishment of fine friendships.

The secret of social success lies in the realisation that every human being has a sense of strangeness in the presence of another human being. Our social education is so deficient, that all but a few robustly normal individuals shrink at making contacts with their fellows without the benefit of a formal introduction. Fear reigns everywhere. If you can break through this icy wall of fear, in ninety-nine cases out of a hundred the stranger will be more than willing to make friends with you. If you but make the gesture of approach, he will meet you more than half way! Do not forget, the stranger is just as afraid of you as you are of him. Like you, he also wants to be certain that you are not going to tear his mask from him, that you are not going to jolt him out of the ego-equilibrium he has so laboriously built up for himself. If you are wise you will signal your good will before he has a chance to doubt it.

Come forward with a smile, with a friendly gesture, with a sense of your own self-esteem, and an easy sureness of manner. This is the best guarantee of a good reception you can give to a stranger. Break the ice by throwing down the weapons of reserve. You make an almost inaudible sound. I have called it " making a noise like a human being ". This imaginary sound is made by the whole body. No musical instrument can reproduce it, and no physicist can test it in a laboratory. It is one of those sounds that you have to hear to appreciate. Once you have learned to " make a noise like a human being " the rest is easy. And remember, the cleverer person makes the first step!

CREATIVE SELF-REALISATION

Perhaps you are one of the people who has no difficulty in making social contacts. You can pick up a conversation with the corner policeman, your neighbour at a concert, or a fellow visitor at an art museum. You fail, not in making contacts, but in following them up. This is the second step in building up a social life, and it is just as important as the first. The world made up of staccato social contacts is empty and void. Many men can make a good impression, but as soon as they have made the first contact they never see their new acquaintances again. To this end you must go out of your way once more. You must invite the stranger with whom you have made the contact to dine with you, to go to another concert, to walk with you in the park, to visit a cinema or theatre, or to meet some other friends of yours. One of the beauties of Continental life is the institution of the café which makes the development of such acquaintances much simpler. But with a little good will and effort they can be made under any conditions. Where the knowledge of the importance of developing acquaintances exists, and the will to practise it has been stimulated by the realisation of its value, ways and means are not hard to find.

These kindergarten exercises in social relations are included in this manual, because in my experience there are a great many men and women whose training has left them utterly unprepared for the amenities of social life. It must not be thought that these preliminary exercises are really the goal of what I call the good social life. They are necessary first steps in the social *gradus ad parnassum*. If you have already learned these first exercises, I know you will pardon me for including them for the guidance of some perplexed brother who has not enjoyed your social advantages. We come now to the real purpose of these preliminary exercises. Each and every one of us must build up a system of social contacts and relations, preferably outside our immediate family life, which will give us an objective basis for sensing our usefulness to our fellow men.

In this way we may support our sense of " face " on the only valid foundations that are available. It is a fundamental law of psychology that we must find our vital focus outside ourselves.

The finer your intellectual training or the greater your technical ability, the wider the scope of your social responsibility must be. Nervous breakdown is no respecter of persons. If you are a bank clerk or a neglected typist, your sphere of social usefulness may be limited to furthering the social activities of your church or club. If you have had greater opportunities, I expect you to take the spirit of these discussions and apply them to your situation. You may find your value by beginning a little theatre movement in your town, or you may make your personality felt by joining some society whose object is civic betterment. Perhaps the tremendously important task of adult education will enlist your active support. I do not care much whether you work for the Boy Scouts, the Legal Aid Society, the Association for the Improvement of the Conditions of the Poor, the Charity Organisation Society, your local Chamber of Commerce, or whether you help to introduce slum clearance schemes. It does not matter whether you become a delegate to the League of Nations Conference for the Limitation of Narcotic Drugs, whether you compensate for your nervous breakdown and its underlying egoism by helping to establish child guidance clinics in the schools of your city, or whether you roll bandages for the Red

Cross. But you *must*, if you want to get well, get out of the charmed circle of your own ego, and make some kind of contribution to the welfare of your fellow men. I leave the scope and the content to you. I am interested only in the principle of the thing. To cure yourself you must break down the walls of fear and reserve. You must lose your ego in whole-hearted service to humanity, in order to find yourself with your sense of " face " secure. The paradox of Christ's words, " They that lose their lives shall find them ", is also the paradox of creative self-realisation. The focus of your ego must lie outside the ego and within the circle of humanity if you want to achieve happiness.

The task of creative self-realisation through social activities need not have an international scope. At the same time that you are beginning your wider social service, you can begin to be more interested in those who occupy your immediate social environment. I mean by this that you can occasionally give a helping hand to a relative, an employee, a personal maid, a chauffeur, a lift girl, or a junior assistant. Charity and social adjustment both begin at home. You cannot work for humanity at large and be unkind to your neighbours. One of my patients was so impressed with my arguments for the extension of his horizons that he gave up his business (thus putting a great many people out of work) and took himself off to China to be a missionary. In the meantime his wife and children suffered neglect and want, and I was compelled to advise his return to prevent the dereliction of his family. He was very angry at receiving my cablegram, and felt that I had contradicted myself. But it was only his neurotic trick of " lying with the truth ". We cannot be true to humanity at large without applying that truth to our next-door neighbours, our relatives, our servants, and our dogs.

In a grown-up world it is not a question of " either egoism . . . or altruism." You cannot annihilate egoism. What I want you to do is to cultivate an emancipated and enlightened egoism, not an immaculate saintliness. You need not go about in sandals and sackcloth to be a good social human being. Common sense will tell you that one county councillor armed with social vision is worth twenty long-haired soap-box orators armed only with enthusiasm. Here are two psychological axioms. If you seek self-realisation within the confines of your own ego, you will get only symptoms and obsessions for your pains. If you seek a creative self-realisation in the service of your fellow men, you will find not only peace of mind, but often the gratitude and respect of your social community. Mental health, self-realisation, the maintenance of " face ", peace of mind, and good sound sleep are to be found only when you devote your vital energies to the socially valuable task of making this world a better place to live in for your fellow men as well as for yourself.

CHAPTER SEVEN

OF CREATIVE SELF-REALISATION

The Art of Getting On with Yourself—The Art of Using Your Leisure—The Cultivation of a Sense of Humour—The Art of Avoiding Arguments—The Art of Living in the Present—On Romantic Illusions—The Art of Being Grown-Up—Clarification and Cure

THE ART OF GETTING ON WITH YOURSELF.

IF you have a nervous breakdown it is very likely that you fall into one of two categories: either you cannot get on with people, or you cannot get on with yourself. Your nervous breakdown is a declaration of bankruptcy in one, sometimes in both, of these important spheres of human activity. I've been trying to explain how important it is for you to find creative self-realisation in the service of your fellow men. It is no less important to get on with yourself if you want to get well. The fact that you have so many symptoms is not only a sign that you have been psychologically " knocked out " by the force of some critical shock. It also shows that you have not developed your inner resources, the kingdom of God that lies within you.

In each and every one of us there is latent a spark of divine creative power. Your own nervous breakdown is an exquisite creation, a new, original, well-thought-out solution of the difficult problem. In another chapter I explained to you why the nervous breakdown was bad art. Its goal is wrong, and therefore, no matter how good your nervous breakdown is (as nervous breakdowns go), it is a useless, painful, and undesirable product of your creative urge. Just as the nervous breakdown is based on fear, ignorance, and mis-education, so also your sense of your inability to create something valuable is based on this same unholy trinity. It is vitally necessary for every human being to exercise his creative ability. If you are not just a human vegetable you want to create. You may be afraid to create, either because you fear ridicule or because you fear that you cannot excel. You may hesitate because you want to secure your sense of " face " on the neurotic premise of pre-eminence, even in creative work. But the need of creating something is greater to-day than it ever has been in the past.

Since the day when men emerged into what we call civilisation there has been a very interesting evolution going on in men's lives. We value human life more highly than ever before in history, because we have realised that the happiness and security of any individual depends largely on the happiness and security of all. As man's regard for human life grew, a parallel growth in man's interest in health and medicine took place.

To-day we can confidently say that our individual

expectancy of life has been enormously increased by medical science. Never before in the history of the world did a baby born into this world have as good a chance to live out his allotted span of three score and ten years. Medicine and public health, both magnificent examples of the technique of self-realisation through service to humanity, have increased your individual expectancy of life, too.

Engineers, working side by side with doctors, have simultaneously found their creative self-realisation by lightening the burden of man's work through the invention of labour-saving devices. Adam wept at his expulsion from Paradise, and his sons resented the necessity of tilling the soil and tending their flocks. They did not know how to harness the forces in nature. In those days men truly ate their bread by the sweat of their brows. Science and invention have made that daily task less and less difficult, until to-day it is confidently stated that if every adult between the ages of twenty-five and forty-five were to work hard for four hours a day, two days a week, the whole work of the world would be accomplished, and every human being could live in comparative luxury and ease.

You are the inheritor of the scientific legacies of the doctors, biologists, and engineers. You not only have more days to live than your ancestors, but you need never work as hard nor as long as they did. This signifies only one thing: the older you grow the more and more leisure you are going to have on your hands, and you will have more and more time to spend by yourself. In addition to the problems of social adjustment, sexual adjustment, and occupational adjustment, science has handed you a new problem: the problem of what to do with your leisure.

Once before in the history of the world this problem presented itself in much the same way. That was in the Golden Age of Greece. In those far-off days all the work of the world was done by unfortunate slaves. The Athenian citizen did not soil his hands. Our machines work for us much more efficiently than the Athenian slaves worked for the gentlemen of Athens, but they leave us with the same problem that faced the Athenians. Do you know what our word 'school' is derived from? It is derived from the Greek word which means spare time, leisure. The Greeks developed their schools to solve their problem of leisure and to keep themselves from being bored to death. I am sure that if we had the records we could find a great many examples of nervous breakdown among the gilded Athenian youths. Satan no doubt found mischief for their idle hands to do, just as he does to-day. Mischief is the work of idle hands; nervous breakdown is the work of the mind at mischief.

What are you going to do with this spare time? I doubt whether you have a creative hobby, because a man with a creative hobby can usually keep from having a nervous breakdown. One of my friends lost his fortune, his child, his wife, and his father within a period of eight months. Certainly this is enough misfortune to rock a very strong person. But he had a wonderful hobby. He was an inveterate archæologist, and when misfortune came to him he gathered together what little remained of his funds, worked his way on a freight steamer to Peru, offered his services to the Peruvian Government, and spent a year fruitfully excavating Inca monuments. That year of research kept him sane and healthy, and enabled him to return home ready to face the problem of beginning his whole life over again at the age of forty.

THE ART OF USING YOUR LEISURE

Hobbies and avocations will not, in themselves, cure a nervous breakdown. But they help immensely. And one of the first things you have to do is to get a hobby. Of course I would prefer your finding a hobby in some field of activity which would incidentally contribute to human happiness. I think that making fine pottery is a better hobby than playing bridge, and I feel that the cultivation of a beautiful garden is a more valuable hobby than doing cross-word puzzles. But both bridge and cross-word puzzles are eminently respectable hobbies. So is stamp collecting, especially if you do it with an eye to historical developments as depicted in your stamps. The true stamp collector will always find at least one young boy to initiate into the mysteries and marvels of philately. Whether you breed Siamese cats, police dogs, or silver foxes, whether you grow an interesting cactus garden, hobbies that have to do with living things are better as a rule than hobbies that have to do only with inanimate objects. Games like chess and bridge have the advantage of being social as well as recreational, and physical sports have the advantage of combining hygienic development with their leisure-solving propensities.

The creative arts, painting, drawing, sculpture, craftsmanship, pottery, literature, the dance, drama, and music are in many senses the ideal hobbies because they set problems which are never finished. There is something about a mass of clay or a piece of marble which offers a challenge to the human spirit, and gives the man who accepts it the most magnificent sense of reality. In my private practice and in my clinic I insist that every patient develops a creative hobby. The more socially valuable your hobby is the better, but the chief criterion of the value of a hobby is this: can it help you over those long hours that you must spend with yourself? It must challenge your creative ability, and it must give you a set of problems that cannot be finished in a day.

There is no reason why you should not develop more than one hobby. If you are troubled chiefly by physical symptoms, due, as I have explained, to imbalances in the vegetative nervous system, a sport will be more beneficial than a purely intellectual hobby. Swimming and rhythmic dancing are excellent for younger individuals, golf and riding are better suited to those in middle age, walking is the cheapest sport, ski-ing one of the most thrilling for those who have the time and money to travel to places where they can enjoy it.

There is no end to the number of available hobbies, and I know there is one that just suits your needs and your temperament. It makes no difference whether your hobby is tinkering with your motor-car or building model aeroplanes, whether you keep bees or do dry-point etchings, whether you decipher Aztec inscriptions or climb mountains, whether you collect Georgian silver or Picasso paintings, whether you read travel books or compose cantatas, whether you tinker with wireless sets or invent household gadgets, whether you do *petit point* or design millinery, whether you paint lampshades or read to the blind. Your hobby is an essential investment in creative self-realisation, and the more hobbies you have, the more interest you take in them—provided you do not lie with the truth and make the business of being an artistic dilettante a goal in life—the better it will be for you.

Do I hear objections? Did I hear you say that you didn't know which hobby to choose? That you have never had a hobby, and would not know how to go about getting one? And did I hear you say that you had no talent for any creative work? And that there was no use taking up the piano because there were already so many outstanding pianists? Let us take up that last objection first. You do not have to be a virtuoso to enjoy a hobby. The idea that people have to be talented, or must be geniuses to create or perform, is one of the most bewhiskered fallacies ever perpetrated on a discouraged world by discouraged neurotics. Time was when it was considered evidence of talent to be able to read. Now everyone can read and write. Do you know that as outstanding a man as Charlemagne could not read or write because one of his instructors said that he didn't have the talent for it?

Nowadays our methods of teaching have improved so much that everyone can learn almost anything that he wants to learn. Not thirty years ago we believed that it required a divine talent to drive a car. Now any schoolboy can drive one. For hundreds of years people believed that women did not have the talent to practise medicine. To-day, in Russia, three-fourths of the practising physicians are women. The fact that you cannot play the piano like Rachmaninoff or Paderewski is no reason for not sitting down and amusing yourself by working out a simple Bach prelude and fugue. You do not have to be a Michelangelo to get a world of pleasure from modelling your cook's head or your dog. No one wants you to be a genius. I want you to have a good time doing something more interesting than broadcasting your symptoms.

As for the choice of a hobby—I have already listed quite a few available ones, and if you use your ingenuity, those mentioned will suggest others to you. Then you can use this question as a means of establishing social contacts. Go round to all your friends and ask them what their hobbies are, and request that they demonstrate them to you. Anyone with a hobby is always willing to tell you about it. If you have no friends, ask the first ten people who pass your door, or the members of your club or church. Take the cross-word puzzle in this evening's newspaper, and begin to work it out. Time yourself, and let us see whether you can become a virtuoso in cross-word puzzles. And if the worst comes to the worst, write a play or a novel about yourself, and how you cured your nervous breakdown. And by the way, thinking about your hobby, or how you are going to choose a hobby, is an excellent way to put yourself to sleep at night.

THE CULTIVATION OF A SENSE OF HUMOUR

The next step in the development of your creative self-realisation is the cultivation of a sense of humour. A sense of humour is the rarest of all human virtues. Sense of humour is really something of a misnomer, because the term is confused so frequently with the ability to laugh or to tell a good story. A sense of humour implies a sense of perspective. It means the ability to laugh at yourself, and still go on doing the best you can in an admittedly imperfect world. Neurotics have no sense of humour, because the sense of humour is the antithesis of their " all or none " philosophy of life. They see themselves as gods in battle with an unkind world, or as worms, trodden by the destroying heel of an unsympathetic humanity. You are neither a god nor a worm. You are a human being, and as such you must cultivate a sense of humour as a saving grace. The ability to laugh at yourself is one of the things that distinguishes you from the lower animals.

One of the best methods of cultivating a sense of humour is to go outside on a clear night and look at the constellation of Andromeda. In this constellation you will see a wisp-like little cloud of stars which astronomers tell us is the great spiral nebula of Andromeda. Light travels through space at the rate of 186,000 miles a second. Travelling at this stupendous speed it takes light, piercing through the cosmic void from the spiral nebula, 900,000 years to reach our little earth! The figures are staggering. The human mind cannot really comprehend them, so magnificent are they in their scope. That flickering beam of light that you see to-night started from those incandescent stars almost a million light years ago! It gives us something to think about.

Think of it! You are reading this book in a room which is many times your size. And yet that room is just an infinitesimal speck in your town or city.

But that city, in turn, is just an insignificant speck on the map. Even if you live in London, you, your room, your borough, your city, could be dropped into the depths of the Atlantic Ocean without being missed. And the Atlantic Ocean occupies but a small portion of our globe, and our whole earth, in turn, is but an infinitesimal speck in our own solar system. And that solar system would be practically invisible to the eye of some imaginary dweller in the spiral nebula of Andromeda, 900,000 light years away at the other end of the cosmos! Can you tell me what difference it makes whether your heart is fluttering, or whether you have an inferiority complex, or whether you have a splitting headache?

Does it seem worth while to spend all that time nurturing your symptoms? Don't you think that you are giving an exaggerated importance to your fears and anxieties? New worlds are being born in the seething cosmic maelstroms, and you can think only of your nervousness!

I know what you are thinking. The cosmos may be very big, and you may be very small compared with it. But at this moment your fear is the most important thing in the cosmos. Yes, my friend, I have heard that objection before. But since things are as they are, it is unlikely that the grand strategy of evolution, that the marvellous and harmonious music of stellar movements, or even the rhythmic processes of our own little world, are going to stop and listen to your complaints. Life is short, but time is very, very long. You have a certain span of years yet to live. You might as well live in harmony with nature. Here is one place where your private logic cannot be carried out. You have succeeded in deceiving yourself. Perhaps you have deceived your family; you may even have deceived your whole community. You cannot deceive nature. You might just as well laugh it off, and get into step!

THE ART OF AVOIDING ARGUMENTS

One of the best ways to develop your sense of humour is to make up your mind that most of the arguments and anxieties that shorten your life and raise your blood-pressure unnecessarily are useless. You have attempted to bolster your "face" by always trying to be right. This has put you into useless conflict with your family and your associates. If you develop a sense of humour you will see that "being right" is one of the most useless things in the world. Suppose you are right. To-morrow science may prove that you are dead wrong. It will be small comfort to know that you were right yesterday at the cost of losing a friend. Or you argue about the truth. What is true at 9.15 to-night will be quite false at 6.45 next Thursday. Truth is relative. The moral virtues of to-day were the sins of your grandparents, and your grandchildren are likely to regard to-day's virtues with the same amused condescension that you bestow on horsehair sofas and marble-topped washstands.

In order to enliven your sense of humour I suggest that you remove from your vocabulary the words of finality, like " absolutely ", " surely ", " always ", " never ", " completely ", " indubitably "," irrevocably ", " inexorably ", and the like. In your conversation substitute those more human words, " nearly ", " relatively ", " almost ", " frequently ", " rarely ", " approximately ", for the godlike words of finality. Demonstrate your sense of humour by teaching your tongue to say " I do not know ", " as it seems to me now ", " according to my limited experience ", " as the facts seem to indicate ", and the like. Your opinions are likely to have more weight if in expressing them you do not tread on your opponent's inferiority complex by opening your remarks with " You're absolutely wrong ", or " Don't be an idiot, I tell you that . . ." It is better to say, " I do not doubt that in many cases your opinion would be valid, but it seems to me that in this particular case, which may be an exception, the facts appear to be . . ."

Do not forget that you are not the only person who likes to play God at some time or another. When two actors, playing God, meet in the same temple, there is usually friction and conflict. *You* do not have to cure the other actor of his delusions. Leave that to nature and to the psychiatrists. Avoid arguments, dissension, futile discussions, and personal quarrels as you would avoid venomous snakes. You do not have to bolster your sense of " face " by proving everyone in the world to be wrong. You do not have to be right all the time. Discretion is the better part of valour when it comes to arguments. Perhaps you do not know when to assert yourself and your human rights, and are afraid you will be trampled into a deeper sense of inferiority by more self-confident individuals? Here is a good rule to use. If the outcome of the argument in which you are engaged will not make the slightest difference to humanity in twenty-five years, don't argue.

THE ART OF LIVING IN THE PRESENT

The fact that you have a nervous breakdown indicates one thing rather definitely. You are either too much concerned with the past and its mistakes, or with the future and its dangers. In either case, or in both, you are not living in the present. You are deferring your life, and this is one of the most dangerous things that you can be doing at this particular time. The past is dead. Ghosts cannot hurt you. The future never comes. As we have said, ninety-nine and forty-four hundredths per cent of the things you have been afraid of have never happened. Worrying will not stop acts of God and the public enemy. Remorse for the past and worry about the future are among the most futile activities that the human brain can conceive. What has happened in the past may explain your present sorry state, but it cannot compel you to remain in it. Look at it in this way: your mistakes in the past have compelled your present difficulties. Living rightly in the present will just as surely determine your future happiness. Your job is in the present, to do now what you have been deferring all your life.

Live dangerously! You have been so interested in being perfectly safe and having your sense of "face" so impregnably secure, that you have foregone every opportunity of extending your enjoyment of life. Take a chance! Have you wanted to go abroad? Take the next train that you can, even if you have to travel third all the way and go steerage on the boat. Have you wanted to take music lessons? Seek out a teacher to-day, and get to work. No matter what people say, apply my precepts about arguments to the matter of Mrs. Grundy's opinion. People will tell you that you have no talent for this, and are too old for that, and that it is too late to begin a new life, that you cannot teach an old dog new tricks! This applies only to cowards. There has never been a significant discovery in science or philosophy which was not berated by Mrs. Grundy. Remember people laughed at Bach, Galileo, Columbus, Pasteur, Edison, the Wright brothers, Lenin, and Einstein. They remained to cheer and pay homage to the men who did the thing that "couldn't be done"!

"It's too late now, Doctor! If I had known you ten years ago I could have taken your advice. You would have changed my whole life!" How often I have heard those defeatist words! *It is not too late, if you want to get well.* You may put off taking my common-sense advice until to-morrow. No matter. You will get well one day later. You may put it off for a week. That means one more week of symptoms and anguish. You may put it off for a year, for ten years. When you follow the dictates of common sense you will get well. Your job is in the present. You have made a sorry mess of things doing them your way in the past. You know of no better way in the future. Take a chance! *Act as if* it were possible to get well, to be happy, by taking my advice in the present. You cannot wipe out the past, and you cannot foretell the future. You *can* live dangerously in the present. Begin now!

ON ROMANTIC ILLUSIONS

Infantile romanticism is one of the chief causes not only of nervous breakdowns but also of human unhappiness. The history of human stupidity is the history of the conflict between romanticism and objective realism. When the savage is frustrated by the perversity of nature, he attempts to compel nature to do his will by the use of magical rite and ritual. When the modern man is frustrated by the same natural force, he applies the same magic, but he dresses that magic in modern clothes, and calls it romanticism. Strip romanticism of its sentimental coverings, and you have the primitive wish-thinking of the Australian aborigine. The psychological process is the same.

Romanticism begins in childhood. The little girl puts on her mother's high-heeled shoes and long dresses, and becomes a Lady. The little boy, caught in the toils of an infantile inferiority complex, puts on his father's tall silk hat, sticks his father's gold-headed cane under his arm, and sallies forth, a Man. Here is primitive magic in its simplest form. Romanticism is nurtured on fairy tales and the wish-thinking of folk-lore and fable. " Day dreaming " is a reality to the child. The romanticism of the nursery is weaned on the comic strips of the daily newspapers. The sentimentality of the cinema and the Sunday School, and the organised deceit of the classroom are its breakfast food! The romantic fallacy achieves its maturity in the teachings of our universities, and it is worshipped at Board meetings of Big Business organizations. The decisions of some judges, and occasionally the acts of Parliament, are its flower. Finally, it is engraved on our tombstones in gilded letters.

The plague of infantile romanticism penetrates every cranny of modern life. Probably the completely mature individual, the man who tries to meet reality objectively in every situation, does not exist. He is a fiction, an ideal norm which we construct to guide us on our way. We are all infected with the virus of romanticism in some department of our lives. If we are realists in the majority of instances, and allow ourselves whimsicalities only in unimportant matters, we are likely to be rather human and interesting people. But if we are predominantly romanticists, we are liable to personality disaster at any moment. Romanticists are for ever wishing that things were otherwise. Like Micawber, they hope that something will turn up which will save them from the consequences of their unreasonable behaviour. Infantile romanticists have an unhappy lot because they are slaves of their own magical arts. Trading with destiny, bargaining with fate, making votive offerings to good fortune, and punishing recalcitrant and malevolent deities make up their entire lives.

Were we living in an age of miracles and fairy tales come true, infantile romanticism would be a very respectable and honourable strategy of life. Those who could wish hardest would be happiest. Instead of tilling the soil and working machines, we would spend our time propitiating gods and goddesses to our advantage. Unfortunately, the fairy-tale era has vanished with the lost continent of Atlantis. We live in an age of realism. The most realistic men and women seem to be the happiest. They do not waste their time petitioning the stars nor punishing the unkind gods. Theirs is a calm and joyous existence, devoid of the ecstasy of the romanticist, it is true, yet protected withal from the terror, the frenzy, the frustrated rage of the disappointed necromancer whose magic has failed.

The romanticist wishes, hopes, and prays. The realist thinks, reasons, and acts. The romanticist leans on his gods and weeps on the bosoms of his goddesses. The realist believes in himself, and enjoys his independence. To the romanticist all things must be perfect. The realist knows that perfection is a fiction, and is satisfied if there are only a few pieces of kidney in the beef-steak pudding. To the romanticist, dreams are always preferable to actualities because he knows only dreams and wishes. To the realist, realities are more interesting than dreams. The realist dreams only to find new uses for his facts.

When the romanticist succeeds, he praises his magic; when he fails he blames his evil stars. When the realist fails he blames his poor technique, and perseveres until he betters it to the point where it brings him a measure of success. The romanticist lives in the memory of the past and the promise of the future. The realist sweats in the present and gets his enjoyment from living. The romanticist is superstitious, gullible, easily elated and discouraged, suspicious of the new, hostile to change, orthodox in belief, and traditionally minded. He is the apostle of feelings, of subjectivity. The realist is rational, sceptical, slow to become enthusiastic, equally slow to become discouraged, cordial to progress and to change, scientifically minded, and heterodox in belief. He is the champion of reason, of objectivity.

Romanticism is more or less normal in childhood. Realism is the concomitant of mental and emotional maturity. When a romantic spirit dominates an adult body, trouble lies ahead. The infantile adult stubbornly refuses to grow up or to relinquish his infantile reactions. Romanticism is often beyond the reach of reason or logic because it is not a function of the intellect, but the result of the persistence of infantile emotional reactions. A university professor can be just as much of a romanticist as a programme seller in a theatre. Growing up is the process of becoming emotionally mature. Growing up is the result of psychological clarification. Psychological clarification can come only from the *conscious* mobilisation of the emotions. Sometimes this process of clarification is the result of a terrific shock. A critical event may serve to throw the spotlight on a false strategy of living, but usually clarification occurs after you have learned to see your own life's pattern with the objective eyes of a friendly but impersonal counsellor.

THE ART OF BEING GROWN-UP

Do you like to show off, make a big impression, hold the limelight, be pre-eminent, be first, wear the newest clothes, have the most money, drive the fastest car, belong to the local 'county', see your name in the society column? If you do, you are an infantile romanticist. Does it annoy you if your neighbour has a bigger house than you have, or do you feel ashamed because you lack a University education? Does the fact that your friend has a larger diamond than you have anger you? Do you think you have been discriminated against? Do you think that people talk about you behind your back? And do you care vitally what they say about you? Are you proud of your good looks, your physique, your ancestry or your membership of the best club? Do you spend a great deal of time on your personal toilet? Is your family's opinion of you more important than the world's? Do you hunt literary "lions"? Do you boast about your golf scores or your son's scholastic attainments to all your friends? Do you believe in astrology, or do you go to gypsy fortune tellers? Do you ever go to a concert just to be seen? And do you subscribe to charities simply because you are afraid your neighbours will talk about you? Are you an inveterate "first nighter"? All these are forms of romantic infantilism, and, as such, they are undesirable traits which may lead to personality disaster at some time or other.

Romanticism in personal and sexual relations is so common that it is often accepted as "normal". Do you believe that "falling in love" is a necessary prerequisite of a happy marriage? Do you believe that your wife, or husband, *owes* you love and respect? Do you think all women are inferior? Do you think that men can never be trusted? Do you feel that opinions of older people should always be deferred to? Is it your feeling that children should be seen and not heard? Do you feel that children should obey their parents implicitly? Would you refuse to marry a girl if you learned that she was no longer a virgin? Do you feel that adultery is an absolute sin? Is it your honest feeling that a man may be excused for extra-marital sexual escapades, but that a woman who "breaks the sanctity of the home" is morally lost? If you are a woman, would you rather be a man? If you are a man, do you think women get all the best in life? If you answer yes to these questions, which apply to your sex, you are an infantile romanticist, and your beliefs may sooner or later involve you in a critical situation in which you will be compelled to save your "face" by having a nervous breakdown.

The fundamental romantic fallacy is the belief that these infantile rites and dogmas are the royal road to happiness. The romanticist looks at happiness as if it were a *thing*. He believes, having been educated in the romantic tradition, that happiness, success, honour and social esteem are his God-given right. When he does not achieve happiness, he naturally feels that he has been cheated of his birthright, and protests violently. In a world of realists his is a voice crying in the wilderness. The fact that the realistic world is apathetic to his rage and his complaints only corroborates the romanticist's belief that he is in the wrong place. He flees from reality, and finds his escape in the world of fantasy, of dreams, of irrationality, of wish-thinking, of make-believe and of magic. He abjures training, logic, reason, and insight. The more you attempt to lure him out of the ivory tower of his romantic isolation, the more he reiterates his romantic credo, and the harder he practises his idealistic necromancy. The more you feed him with logic, the harder he dreams.

There is a very practical side to the discussion of infantile romanticism. Romanticism does not pay in the end. It leads inevitably to personality disasters. Probably you, too, have believed hard in one of the romantic fictions, only to have come to grief. Your nervous breakdown may be directly traceable to an intolerable conflict between your romantic ideas of "face" and the objective demands of a real world. Why not make your farewells to the house of youth, gracefully and in good time, and matriculate in the house of maturity? Let us say good-bye to the romantic fictions and beliefs, and begin living by reason rather than by wishes and dreams. Happiness is not your birthright. It is not a thing, not a blue bird that you can capture by assiduous search. It is a quality of the good life, and an attribute of realistic living. No one owes you happiness. Human beings may achieve happiness by an honest investment in the good life.

Happiness is an attribute of the application of a realistic technique to the art of living.

Begin now to remove as many of your romantic ideas and actions as possible from your strategy of living. Reality is much more interesting than romance. You would not see scientists spending long years in research if realism did not have its rewards in happiness. A man who builds a house builds happiness, a man who builds a "castle in Spain" builds only disappointment. I would rather write this small book than day-dream about writing a magnificent encyclopædia of psychology. Count that day well spent when you have explored some corner of the vast *terra incognita* of reality, and count that day lost which you have spent only in day-dreaming of grandiose accomplishments.

The fear that romanticists have of reality is based on their ignorance. Listen to your wireless. Is not the miracle of reality more marvellous than the miracle of the dream or the magic of the wish? Look at the electric light bulb. Is not the magic of that light more fascinating than all the will-o'-the-wisps of fantasy? Feel this little book. Hundreds of realists have contributed to its making, so that you and I, separated perhaps by thousands of miles of land and sea, could spend these moments of spiritual contact together. These pages, made possible only by the objective contributions of generations of realists, bring you my experience, my sympathy, and my words of encouragement. They have enabled us to talk as if you were seated in my study. Perhaps some word, some phrase, some example has stirred you to fresh courage, and has contributed to that inner clarification which will be the beginning of your happiness. That, my friend, is the romance of realism; and it is incomparably more thrilling than all the day-dreams of a century!

CLARIFICATION AND CURE

You have been like an engineer challenged by a great project. You have had to build a bridge across an abyss, and your happiness depended on your ability to build it. You wanted it to be strong and beautiful. You have tried to build the bridge and failed. You have been discouraged, you have lost hope, you have questioned the value of the whole project. Your plans failed; your materials were found wanting. The harder you tried, the more perplexing your results became. You knew something was wrong, but you did not know where your chief difficulties lay. Your family and your friends criticised you. In your confusion you ran away from the problem, but your conscience would not let you hide. You made excuses for your failure, and although you began to believe your own excuses, you sensed that they were just excuses, and not real reasons for the failure. In your realisation that something was basically wrong, you turned to this book for expert guidance.

The realisation of your difficulties and your decision to seek help were, as I have already said, the beginning of clarification, and clarification is more than half the cure of your difficulties. In the foregoing pages you learned much that will be valuable in your new attack on your project. You discovered that your failing was not unique. You learned, moreover, that your nervous breakdown, far from being an index of hopeless incompetence, was a very excellent compromise between your own poor preparation for the task and the demands of the difficult project you have had to solve. In other words, you have already built a skeleton bridge across your abyss, but you know that it will not stand the strain, nor come up to the specifications of the contract.

At this point we must issue an important reservation. There are certain cases which will not be cured by the application of the principles outlined in this book. In some of these cases the nervous breakdown is a practically effective bridge between the patient's inner constitution and the demands of a neurotic environment, and the patient is unable to change his environment. In other cases the inner conflicts are so deeply hidden in the unconscious that they are not accessible to the patient himself, and the practice of conscious attempts at normal activity cannot entirely solve the patient's activities. These are the cases where a prolonged psychological analysis and re-education at the hands of a qualified psychiatrist are required to give insight and clarification to the patient. If you have carried out the instructions in this book to the best of your ability, over some period of time, and no relief is obtained, I counsel you to put yourself in the care of a reputable psychiatrist and undergo the process of psychological re-education, no matter how great the sacrifice in time and money may be. Under these circumstances you cannot afford *not* to avail yourself of psychiatric help.

I hope you are one of those readers who has learned the true nature of his difficulties for the first time through these pages. Clarification is still almost wholly an intellectual process for you. You have analysed your mistakes, your mis-education, your ignorance of the task before you, your ineffectual responses. In the past, your satisfying emotions have been attached to the wrong actions. In the past you have enjoyed only subjective experiences, and have usually disliked socially useful acts. We must now re-educate your emotions so that you will enjoy socially constructive conduct, and dislike the egoistic, self-aggrandising, self-defending, isolating behaviour which has resulted in your nervous breakdown. The practical suggestions in the foregoing pages were written especially for you. You must now make the investment in normal living. You must now break down the walls about your self and find a focus for your vital activities outside the charmed circle of your own ego. You must begin to make contributions to your fellow men. I know that it is not easy for you, because your whole training militates against this new course of conduct that I have outlined for you. Do not be afraid. After all, your situation could not be greatly aggravated by following common-sense counsel. These instructions, if properly carried out, will help you to ameliorate your situation at the very least. The most they can do is to cure your nervous breakdown, completely, and for all time.

You will make objections, to be sure, to this and to that specific piece of advice. You will tell me that my instructions do not fit your particular case, temperament, training, or opportunities. Try to apply as much of my counsel as you can, and while you are applying it new methods and new techniques will spontaneously suggest themselves to you. You need only remember the broad outlines—the details are part of your own task of creative self-realisation. Do not expect brilliant or immediate results. If you put your money in the savings bank on Friday afternoon, you cannot expect to get much interest on your money on Saturday morning. The same applies to the process of curing yourself of your nervous breakdown.

As it is, you will probably be amazed at the results. You will awaken one fine morning, and that dull, tired feeling will be gone. You will find yourself sleeping eight hours a night, without taking pills to make you sleep. People will begin to notice that your expression has changed and that you look much happier. The tasks ahead of you will seem less fearsome. You will notice that more people in your environment are smiling. You will find that it is not difficult to eat like other people, and that you do not have to maintain that strict diet you have been keeping. Your dreams will be more encouraging. One day you will find yourself doing something constructive and you will say to yourself, "I could never have done that before!" And the process of creative self-realisation will be under way.

When you will have finished this book, you will have realised that your nervous breakdown is not an accident and not a sickness in the sense that measles or diphtheria are sicknesses. Your nervous breakdown is a compromise between your inner urges and instincts and the problems of the external world which you, as a citizen of that world, must solve as well as possible. But your nervous breakdown is a socially unacceptable compromise. It is obvious, therefore, that you are not going to be cured by pills, by diet, by sexual relations, by surgical operations, by rest cures, sea voyages, or a change of air. You must know the truth, you must mobilise your conscious efforts to obtain a better understanding of your problems, and, with the aid of your new insight, you must find a more effective strategy of solving them, and greater courage and perseverance in your attack. Cure can come in only one way: the conscious re-direction of your vital energies to the attainment of a goal that not only satisfies your primitive urges, instincts, and desires, but also serves to maintain your sense of " face " by winning social approval for your acts.

You have felt dead and unreal and fatigued because your false strategy of life has met with frustration on all sides. You must cultivate the thrill of aliveness, get into step with the throbbing rhythm of reality, and find the physical well-being that comes with confidence and success, by risking a new attack. Remember you are better armed than ever before. These pages have not only helped you to analyse your former failures. They have also given you a new and dependable map of the battlefront of reality, and indicated a technique and strategy that has been found good in hundreds of similar situations. The sense of deadness, of unreality, of hopeless fatigue that you have experienced is the result of only one thing: an inefficient and unconstructive utilisation of your vital energies and reserves.

Both your body and your mind are so constructed that you are the master of almost unlimited powers. Do not give up because you are tired. Get your second wind. You have a third wind, even a fourth wind, if you will but tap your own vital reserves. Think how hard you have been concentrating on your symptoms and your illness! One tenth of that same energy, directed to a useful and socially constructive goal, will bring you incredible dividends in happiness. The first thing to do is to throw away your mental crutches, your physical alibis, excuses, exonerations and self-pityings. Throw all the bottles of medicine that you have been taking out of the window. Forget the diets and the tonics and the sedatives! Life is the best tonic, hard work the best hypnotic ever created, and living itself the best sedative for jangled nerves that man has ever found.

What I hope is that in reading these pages, and in the course of your heart-to-heart talk with me, you may have experienced a sense of inner clarification. It is as if you have been sitting in a dark theatre watching a play on the dimly lit stage. Suddenly a brilliant spotlight has illuminated the scene and stage; players and background appear in a new and clearer relationship. What had been a mysterious and unintelligible confusion of voices and actions becomes transformed, as if magically, into a meaningful performance, whose plot, scene, and personalities suddenly acquire reality for you. You have been quietly confessing your mistakes and illusions to me, and in talking with me, you have suddenly discovered the truth yourself. All you really needed was a sympathetic listener. The cure of your difficulties lies within yourself. Clarification is the key which solves the nervous breakdown, but only the sufferer has the key to his own situation. All I have done was to suggest where you might look for the misplaced key. You needed to share your fears and your anxieties with someone whom you trusted. Our conversation has served to convince you that your situation is not hopeless. The dread, the anxiety, the confusion and the perplexity of the last weeks or months has suddenly lifted. You feel re-born. Your head is high, your vision is again keen, your spirit encouraged.

I congratulate you. I know that your experience of clarification will enable you to face your problems with a new courage. I need not urge you to share this encouragement with your fellow men. You have already thought of a friend who needs just the kind of advice and counsel that I have given you, and it will not be long before you find an opportunity to share your new-found knowledge with him. Even now you look back at your former mistaken attitudes and actions as if they were part of a dim and unpleasant dream. The world of reality is much sweeter than it has ever been for you. You are on your way to creative self-realisation.

We have come to the end of my book, and the beginning of your psychological renaissance. Your life begins where my book ends. You have gained insight into your own nature and into the nature of your psychological mechanisms. You know the truth, and the truth has made you free to begin the task of creative self-realisation. It may not go easily in the beginning. Your symptoms may recur, but do not let that hinder your progress. A great philosopher has said, "Every man becomes a Stoic if he lives long enough." Be a Stoic. Grit your teeth at symptoms, and go on. Remember that the pain and the adversity of to-day make your happiness sweeter to-morrow. Throw off the shackles of the past, and don't worry about the future. Live to-day. Live now. I give you courage, hope, and the will to get well!